The Epidemiology of Chronic Digestive Disease

M. J. S. Langman BSc, MD, FRCP
Professor of Therapeutics
University of Nottingham Medical School

An Edward Arnold Publication
Distributed by
Year Book Medical Publishers, Inc.
35 E. Wacker Drive, Chicago

© M. J. S. Langman 1979

First published 1979
by Edward Arnold (Publishers) Ltd
41 Bedford Square, London WC1B 3DQ

All Rights Reserved. No part of this publication may be reproduced, stored in a retrieval system, or transmitted in any form or by any means, electronic, mechanical, photocopying, recording or otherwise, without the prior permission of Edward Arnold (Publishers) Ltd.

Distributed in the United States of America
by Year Book Medical Publishers, Inc.

ISBN 0-8151-5305-8
Library of Congress Catalog Card Number 79-90181

Printed in Great Britain

Preface

Chronic digestive disease is common, it is frequently disabling and, if due to cancer, is seldom curable. Knowledge of its root causes is fragmentary, but is increasing. The available information is scattered through a variety of sources which include epidemiological, clinical and basic scientific journals. This book sets out to provide an overall picture of digestive disease frequency and of the factors which predispose to it. Liberal use has been made of illustrative tables designed to give examples of representative data.

I am grateful to the editors and authors for permission to use figures and tables on pages 22, 82, 44, drawn from *Gut*, the *Scandinavian Journal of Gastroenterology*, and *Science*. I am also grateful to my secretary Mrs. Janice Avery for typing the manuscript. I would have dedicated the book to my teachers, particularly Sir Richard Doll and Sir Francis Avery Jones, for stimulating my interest in the subject, but they deserve something better; or to my wife, but she deserves something different. Lastly I am grateful to my publishers for their patience and help.

Nottingham, 1979   MJSL

Contents

1. **General introduction**   1
   Terminology and descriptive methods
   Incidence rates, prevalence rates and death rates
   Official statistics

2. **Peptic ulcer**   9
   prevalence and incidence; geographical and environmental factors; other factors; associated diseases; genetic factors; psychological factors

3. **Gastrointestinal cancer**   40
   Oesophageal cancer
   Gastric cancer
   Small intestinal cancer
   Large intestinal cancer
   Pancreatic cancer
   Hepatic cancer
   Cancer of the gallbladder and bile ducts

4. **Chronic non-specific inflammatory bowel disease**   80
   Crohn's disease
   Ulcerative colitis
   Factors in common to colitis and Crohn's disease

5. **Diverticular disease and appendicitis**   103
   Diverticular disease
   Appendicitis

6. **Gallstones**   114
   age and sex distribution; time trends; geographical incidence and ethnic variation; diet; predisposing diseases; hereditary factors

7. **Pancreatitis**   129
   Incidence and time trends; geographical trends; nutrition; associated conditions; drug-induced pancreatitis; genetic factors

Index   136

1
General introduction

Gastrointestinal disease is common, yet we have a poor insight into its root causes. Study of the distribution and determinants of individual diseases can yield valuable information about the patterns and behaviour of disease. Much information is already collected in routine statistics, and in understanding what is already available and what can be gained from special surveys and examinations, some simple epidemiological knowledge is required.

Terminology and descriptive methods

The fundamental basis for epidemiological studies is that they describe patients in relation to the population from which they come. Therefore frequency rates can be calculated which relate the number of individuals with a disease to the population from which they are drawn as, respectively, numerator and denominator. These sets of people may be national or regional populations, or some special subgroup according, for instance, to occupation, sex or age.

Incidence rates, prevalence rates and death rates

A critical distinction has to be made between the numbers or proportions of people in a given population who have a disease and the number of new cases arising within a set period. The difference may seem small, but there are likely to be gross variations where a disease persists lifelong.

Incidence rates

These describe the number of new cases arising in a set time period, for a given group of the population, and a convenient figure for chronic disease such as peptic ulcer or gastrointestinal cancer is the number of new cases arising per 100 000 population in a year. Interpretation of a simple figure of this type may still be difficult. Thus if fifty new cases of a disease arise each year per 100 000 population in an area where the population is a quarter of a million, then there will be expected overall to be 125 new cases a year.

2   *General introduction*

Table 1.1 Calculation of standardized incidence rates: Gastric cancer.

Age	Observed incidence per 100 000 population	Standard population	∴ expected cases in standard population
Using a standard population with a lower proportion of elderly people			
0–20	0·0	30 000	0·00
21–40	6·2	40 000	2·48
41–60	40·1	20 000	8·02
61 and over	200·0	10 000	20·00
All ages		100 000	30·50
Using a standard population with a higher proportion of elderly people			
0–20	0·0	30 000	0·00
21–40	6·2	35 000	2·17
41–60	40·1	25 000	10·03
61–80	200·0	15 000	30·00
All ages		100 000	42·20

However, the simple statistics may conceal the fact, as with gastrointestinal cancer, that incidence rises markedly with age. Furthermore there is a commonsense need to consider the reality of the figures. Are all cases ascertained within the area under review? If not, is this because patients fail to present with the disease? Is it because diagnostic fashions vary from place to place? Is it because special centres outside the area under survey collect some of the disease population from the survey area and consequently that disease is under-registered within the area? Is it because the survey method is inappropriate?

Thus, in considering ulcerative colitis within a geographical region, mild cases may fail to present at all, and some cases may be unrecognized even if they do present if medical services are poor. Diagnostic fashion may dictate that the label of Crohn's disease is applied rather than ulcerative colitis; alternatively amoebiasis may be so common that non-specific inflammatory bowel disease goes unrecognized. Finally, if hospital admission statistics are used as a basis of case ascertainment they will undoubtedly miss many cases which are managed solely as outpatients.

Prevalence rates

These describe the number of individuals suffering from a disease at any particular time in a set population. For chronic diseases prevalence rates will be far higher than incidence rates, whereas for transitory illnesses like influenza the prevalence of active disease may, during an epidemic, be lower than the incidence of new cases, arising simply because a disease episode lasts a few days whilst the incidence rate may be calculated for, say, a full month.

Death rates

These may be as useful as incidence rates in measuring the impact of certain diseases where the chances of death from that disease are very high. Thus they can be taken as indicators of disease frequency in most varieties of gastrointestinal cancer, but it would be foolish to do the same with a disease like peptic ulcer where most people do not die.

Standardized rates

Where diseases vary greatly in their age distribution it is necessary to employ some procedure which allows like to be compared with like. Thus, gastric cancer rises in frequency with age and is comparatively common in the United Kingdom. By contrast, it is rare in most tropical areas. Could this difference be simply accounted for by the fact that Western populations contain a higher proportion of elderly people than do most tropical populations? To obtain comparability it is useful either to compare age-specific disease incidence or mortality rates or to standardize for age.

Age specific rates simply confine attention to all cases occurring in people of a set age, say 50 to 55 years, and relate the numerator of the number of diseased individuals to a denominator of the number of people of that age in the population.

Age standardized rates can be derived as single figures for a population of all age groups and are useful in broad comparisons of one group and another. They can be derived by taking age specific rates and applying them to a standard population which has predetermined proportions of individuals of set ages. The methods of calculation used in considering gastrointestinal cancer, and which can equally be applied elsewhere, are given in Table 1.1. Clearly, such a method will compensate for the effects of variations in the distribution of people of different ages in the original population. Equally, the age distribution of the standard population will weight the absolute figure obtained at the end of the calculation. The lower part of the table shows the effect of weighting the standard population with greater numbers of elderly people in considering a disease like gastric cancer which particularly affects the elderly.

4   *General introduction*

Table 1.2 Calculation of standardized mortality ratios: Occupational mortality in Punch & Judy operators.

Number of men by age group	Number of men in population under study	Death rate in the general population per 100 000 per year
15–24	10 000	0
25–34	25 000	1·5
35–44	30 000	10·0
45–54	25 000	50·0
55–64	20 000	200·0

Total observed deaths in occupational population = 102.

Standardized mortality ratio = total number of actual deaths in population under study ÷ the expected number of deaths in each age group if death rates applicable to the general population had applied, multiplied by 100.

$$\text{Expected deaths} = 10\,000 \times \frac{0}{100\,000} + 25\,000 \times \frac{1\cdot 5}{100\,000} + \cdots$$

$$= 0 + 0\cdot 38 + 3\cdot 00 + 12\cdot 50 + 40\cdot 00 = 55\cdot 88$$

$$\therefore \text{SMR} = \frac{102}{55\cdot 88} \times 100 = 183$$

Standardized mortality ratios

Comparisons of the mortality experience of people in different occupations are made more meaningful by taking into account the age of the individuals concerned. The Registrar General's tables in England and Wales employ the standardized mortality ratio (SMR) for this purpose, as do others. Basically the calculation is made by taking the total number of deaths in the people in the occupational category in question and dividing it by the sum of the numbers of men in each age group in that occupation, multiplied by the death rates which would have been obtained if the figures for the general population applied, and then multiplying the whole by 100. Table 1.2 illustrates such a calculation for men aged 15–64 years in an occupation where there is about twice the expected mortality from gastric cancer. It can be seen that by aggregating all deaths from the disease in question in the occupational group under study, the method ignores the random variations with age which can give rise to difficulties of interpretation when numbers in each age group are small. The method can equally be applied to other sub-groups of a population, such as religious groups, as to occupational groups.

Official statistics

The range of official statistics available for scrutiny is wide. The Registrar General publishes an Annual Statistical Review of England and Wales, and periodic supplements on cancer. Equivalent publications are available in many other countries. Sound interpretation demands two cardinal considerations. First, the techniques used in analysis must be examined and understood and second, the methods of collection of data must be considered for their appropriateness.

Mortality data

These have been considered earlier (p. 3). The use of mortality data is seldom helpful in examining secular and other trends in the behaviour of chronic digestive disease because the ratio of deaths to disease incidence is generally low. High death rates from, say, peptic ulcer may be associated with high overall incidence rates, but they may also reflect inadequacies in health care, a tendency for the disease in that area to affect the elderly, differences in the frequency of post mortem examinations or the assiduity with which the examination is conducted or even simply variations in coding practices on death certificates. Such problems do not automatically make mortality statistics valueless to the gastroenterologist, but they emphasize the care with which analyses must be conducted. Even when a disease is, for epidemiological purposes, uniformly fatal, like gastric cancer, care must still be exercised in comparing sets of data.

Death certificates are primarily legal instruments and secondarily sources of information about disease patterns. The accuracy of death certificates is not checked routinely in this country, and substantial errors can arise either through variations in coding practices or from simple errors through clinical mis-diagnosis. Data derived from death certificates are adjusted if the results of post mortem examinations are known and reported, but post mortem examinations are seldom conducted on patients who die outside hospital unless death is sudden and unexpected, and, in England, Wales and possibly elsewhere, the frequency of post mortem examination of patients dying in hospital has fallen, and tends to be especially low in the elderly. Until 1975 the primary cause of death only was coded, this being done, as now, according to the International Classification of Disease published by the World Health Organization. This has changed, and all causes of death given on certificates are now coded so that two or more coincident diseases can be recognized officially as well as clinically.

Occupational mortality The recording of peoples' occupations on death certificates allows figures to be compiled about death rates in different occupations. Roughly every ten years the Registrar General publishes analyses of occupational mortality which include figures for individual occupations, and according to five broad social groups, which are:

Social class I – Higher professional and administrative
II – Intermediate occupations
III – Skilled occupations
IV – Partly skilled occupations
V – Unskilled occupations

These figures are valuable and show large fluctuations, for instance in mortality rates from gastric cancer by social class. Difficulties of interpretation may arise, such as in deciding whether the lower mortality rates which tend to prevail in social classes I and II are due to a greater ability to obtain good medical care than in classes IV and V. In addition the occupation which is coded is the last held by the individual who has died, yet any relevant occupational exposure to health risks may have taken place ten or more years before, when the individual held a different job.

Hospital admission statistics Figures giving the diagnoses of patients admitted to hospital are available in many areas. Thus in England and Wales the Registrar General collects a 10% sample of all discharges and deaths, and publishes a yearly analysis of this Hospital Inpatient Enquiry (HIPE). In addition, details of all hospital admissions are now collected by Hospitals Activity Analysis (HAA) in a survey which overlaps and complements HIPE.

These figures can be used for such purposes as reviewing temporal and geographical patterns of distribution. Much the same precautions must be taken in reviewing such figures as in considering mortality statistics. Though admission or discharge data relate to a far greater proportion of individuals having chronic digestive diseases than do mortality statistics, they cannot be accepted as a random sample of all those actually suffering from the diseases in question. Thus, hospital admissions for peptic ulcer now consist mainly of those with complications of bleeding and perforation or who have had sufficiently persistent or disabling symptoms to justify operation. The assumption that this has always been so would be unjustified; attitudes to the virtues, or probable lack of virtue of courses of inpatient medical treatment coupled with the availability of new potent anti-ulcer drugs has almost certainly reduced the demand for admission, though the scale of the change is hard to determine.

A particular subgroup of individuals with a disease is sometimes used as an index for gauging comparative frequencies from time to time or from place to place. Such figures have their virtues but again, there are possible errors, thus diseases are not necessarily of equivalent severity in different places or at different times.

Sickness returns   Such returns compiled for health insurance purposes can be used to look at disease trends with time, or from place to place. Before accepting such figures at their face value it is essential to consider whether the data are truly comparable. Certificates of disability may have a medical diagnosis attached, but this label is there to give an acceptable reason for illness both to the insurance system and to the doctor and patient. Psychiatric illness may be given a physical disease label, some physical diseases may be currently fashionable and some of the labels, such as gastritis, are so vague as to be almost meaningless. Evidence derived from health insurance data can be taken to support other figures but it is seldom possible to place great reliance on the figures.

Cancer registration   In the United Kingdom, like many other countries, cancer registries have been established. In this country individual hospitals are responsible for registration, and this is generally done by clerical staff and not clinicians. Cancer registration is not a legal necessity and it can be incomplete; likewise disease coding may not be uniform, though this is probably a greater problem with extra-gastrointestinal tumours. The Registrar General sends to individual cancer registries copies of death certificates of patients who are recorded on those certificates as having cancer and who have died in that registry's area.

Special surveys   From time to time surveys are conducted which enquire into specific problems. Apart from those carried out by individuals with interests in certain diseases large scale surveys have been conducted in a variety of situations. The Registrar General has published a series of reports on medical and population subjects, including one on the accuracy of certification of death. In 1955–56 the Royal College of General Practitioners collected records of consultations in a large group of practices throughout the country. In the USA there have likewise been many specific enquiries including Vital and Health Statistics Reports which appear regularly.

Methods of population survey

Cross-sectional surveys   These should identify all individuals who have a disease at a specific time and therefore, if sampling is properly done, should give estimates of disease prevalence. They can also be used to enquire into causative factors by looking back at antecedent features of patients' lives. Such retrospective data are often hard to interpret because patients' opinions about their earlier lives are likely to be coloured by the existence of disease. A further problem is that if patients have certain characteristics it is usually impossible to decide if the disease predisposed to those characteristics or the characteristics predisposed to the disease.

Longitudinal surveys Such a study starts with a survey which defines the initial characteristics of a population including those with disease and those who are disease-free. Subsequently it is possible to measure the incidence of new disease by follow up of those who were initially disease-free, in addition it may be possible to delineate risk factors for disease if the initial survey has included analyses of possible factors. The Framingham study has been used to identify risk factors, such as overweight, for gallbladder disease by examining the incidence of the disease in people who were initially healthy and who, at the start of the survey, had their body weights noted. Longitudinal studies are expensive, time consuming and need clear planning to ensure that enough individuals are included initially for a reasonable number to develop disease later and to include at the start a reasonable range of possible risk factors for later examination.

General references

Alderson, M. (1976). *An Introduction to Epidemiology*. London, MacMillan.

Armitage, P. (1971). *Statistical Methods in Medical Research*. Oxford, Blackwell.

Barker, D. J. P., Rose, G. (1976). *Epidemiology in Medical Practice*. Edinburgh, Churchill Livingstone.

Hill, A. B. (1977). *A Short Textbook of Medical Statistics*. London, Hodder and Stoughton.

MacMahon, B., Pugh, T. F. (1970). *Epidemiology. Principles and Methods*. Boston, Little Brown.

Snedecor, G. W., Cochran, W. G. (1967). *Statistical Methods*. (6th Edition). Iowa State University Press.

2
Peptic ulcer

Peptic ulcer is a general public health problem throughout the world. Statistics from all sources indicate that 10% or more of Western populations may be afflicted by the disease at some time in their lives. Peptic ulcer also accounts for approximately 10% of all adult admissions to general medical and surgical hospitals and for an appreciable proportion of all new cases attending outpatient clinics.

Progress in understanding the predisposing causes of peptic ulcer and its true frequency is hindered by a number of problems. Though there is clear evidence that gastric and duodenal ulcer are different diseases, epidemiological analyses often do not distinguish between them and hence are greatly reduced in value. Even when the distinction is made, there is still considerable difficulty in finding reliable bases for comparison. The sources of information on the incidence of peptic ulcer disease are:

(1) Mortality rates. These are of limited value, because gastric and duodenal ulcers seldom cause death and may well not be noted even if known to be present as ancillary conditions.

(2) Post-mortem surveys. Provided special attention is paid to gastroduodenal examination, such studies can provide much useful information, though few attempts have, in fact, been made.

(3) Clinical statistics. These may provide information about the number of times the disease was diagnosed in relation to the number of hospital admissions or patient visits within a given period of time. However, the hospital population itself may be highly selected, reflecting referral patterns to the hospital and the specialized interests and skills of the hospital staff. Admission with uncomplicated ulcer is relatively infrequent, except for elective surgery, and the criteria for admission for elective medical and surgical treatment probably vary so much that useful comparisons between areas and times can seldom be made. Analyses of complication rates of acute bleeding, and, particularly, perforation are probably more reliable but suffer from the disadvantage that complications only occur in a minority of ulcer patients, and

conclusions reached in these few may not necessarily apply to the majority.

(4) Prevalence and incidence studies. Population survey in a defined locality, where either the whole population or a random sample of a population of known age and sex structure are investigated forms the best method of determining ulcer frequency. Using this method, disease incidence (the number of new cases in a known time interval for a set population) or prevalence (the total number of patients having the disease irrespective of date of diagnosis in a set population) can be measured by, for instance, investigating radiologically all those with significant dyspepsia in whom no search for ulcer has already been made. Such surveys are clearly tedious and time consuming.

Despite all the difficulties, large amounts of data have been collected and show obvious variations in ulcer frequency throughout the world.

Prevalence and incidence

Autopsy studies Though great variations in ulcer frequency have been reported following post-mortem surveys conducted throughout the world, much of this fluctuation can probably be ascribed to the differing criteria applied in judging whether there was evidence of active or previous ulceration. Failure, for instance, to ensure that the duodenal bulb was examined both internally and externally could lead to many ulcers being missed.

Another obvious source of difficulty lies in deciding whether there is or is not significant scarring indicative of past, but now healed ulceration.

Even when these problems are borne in mind it is clear that ulcer can be very common. Watkinson[1] has emphasized the value of data obtained in post-mortem surveys in patients dying suddenly in hospital, or in all hospital deaths when special attention was paid to the routine examination of the stomach and duodenum. He found that in Leeds, England approximately 20% of all men and 10% of women had evidence of present or previous ulcer. Similar high frequencies have been found in Sweden, and also in the Netherlands[2] where nearly a quarter of all patients had evidence of ulcer disease. Table 2.1 illustrates some of these findings. In all such surveys it must be emphasized that the proportion of patients dying of ulcer would in fact be a small fraction of the number found to have evidence of ulcer.

Ulcer mortality Gastric and duodenal ulcer account for a minor proportion of deaths compared with cardiovascular disease and cancer of the digestive and extra-digestive systems, and Table 2.2

Table 2.1 Frequency of peptic ulcer found at necropsy.

	Leeds[1] 1930–49		Rotterdam[2] 1940–59	
	Men	Women	Men	Women
Chronic gastric ulcer				
active	2·4	1·3	8·5	5·6
inactive	1·5	1·6		
Chronic duodenal ulcer				
active	5·5	1·5	10·2	5·4
inactive	6·1	3·3		
Combined ulcer				
active	1·5	0·6	1·1	0·6
inactive	0·8	0·5		
Acute and subacute				
ulcer	2·7	2·2	7·5	6·2
Totals	20·5	11·0	27·3	17·2

Table 2.2 Deaths from peptic ulcer and other causes in England and Wales, 1967.[3]

Peptic ulcer	3 861
Cancer of the stomach	12 936
Malignant disease outside the gut	71 378
Disease of the central nervous system	84 960
Disease of the respiratory system	95 118
Degenerative heart disease	148 869
Deaths from all causes	542 516

illustrates this contrast. The tendency for deaths to be more common in men than women reflects the overall frequency pattern of ulcer, but the tendency for gastric ulcer to be almost as common a cause of death as duodenal ulcer (Table 2.3) is almost certainly due to the tendency for gastric ulcer to affect the elderly, whereas duodenal ulcer is more a disease of middle age.

Ulcer mortality rates vary greatly with socioeconomic status, and these trends are well illustrated by figures obtained in the USA[5] and in the United Kingdom.[6] Poorer people in westernized communities have probably always been more prone to die from gastric ulcer than richer people, but the tendency for poorer people to be prone to duodenal ulcer death as well seems to be a more recent trend.

Table 2.3 Average number of ulcer deaths per 100 000 population, England and Wales, 1968.[4]

		Age 0–44	Age 45–64	Age 65+
Gastric ulcer	Men	2·6	113	613
	Women	1·6	39	419
Duodenal ulcer	Men	3·0	151	812
	Women	0·5	29	268

Mortality is as much a measure of the age distribution of the population with ulcer and of the quality of medical care as of true ulcer behaviour, and therefore it seems preferable to depend upon morbidity statistics as measures of ulcer frequency wherever possible.

Ulcer morbidity and population surveys The best method of assessment would in theory be by population survey, but few such attempts have been made and reliance frequently has to be placed upon simpler clinical statistics such as hospital admission and complication rates. These are cruder measures but they can still emphasize large variations in disease frequency, for instance in different areas of Africa and India where sophisticated analytical methods have not been applied. Table 2.4 compares the reported frequency of ulcer during surveys conducted in various parts of the world. These figures, obtained within areas where ulcer is very

Table 2.4 Frequency detected in some population surveys.

	Frequency percentage		
	Diagnosed ulcer	Likely ulcer	All dyspepsia and ulcer
Australia 1968[7]	7·2	—	—
India, Assam 1968[8]	8·4*	15·1	28·4
Israel[c,9]	8·9*		
United Kingdom			
London 1946[a,10]	5·2*	1·3	31·0
Aberdeen 1961[b,11]	9·9*	5·2	35·2
USA 1965–67[d,12]	2·5*	—	

* Men only
a Questionnaire and clinical and radiological examination where relevant
b Questionnaire, hospital record check and three year follow-up
c Questionnaire, clinical examination and five year follow-up
d Questionnaire alone

common, show a greater degree of uniformity than is generally detectable. Allowance must also be made for the variable methods of survey which were utilized. Thus, the US population survey,[12] which depended upon simple questionnaires designed to detect recent symptomatic disease, is likely to have understated the total frequency of ulcer, whereas the Scottish survey,[11] which combined questionnaire with hospital record analyses and a three year follow-up, should have come closer to assessing the true proportion of individuals with ulcer.

The apparent uniformity of some of these estimates also conceals much variation within and between regions, and Table 2.5 illustrates some of the differences which are detectable when all types of evidence are combined. This will be referred to in more detail later.

Chronological change in incidence The pattern of peptic ulcer frequency has changed greatly in the past century, especially in the age and sex incidence and in the distribution between gastric and duodenal ulcers. During the nineteenth century, gastric ulcer was the predominant lesion and was a particular problem in young women. However at the beginning of this century duodenal ulcer became a defined and important clinical entity, and for the last fifty years has been much more common in most areas than gastric ulcer. The capacity for changes is shown by the male to female ulcer perforation ratio in Scotland after 1920 (Table 2.6). The reasons for this continued alteration are unknown.

Table 2.6 Perforated ulcer in Scotland. Sex-ratios in reported series.

Series	Area	Years of study	Male:Female ratio DU	Male:Female ratio GU
Illingworth et al., 1944[13]	West Scotland	1924–43	21:1	8·7:1
Jamieson, 1955[14]	West Scotland	1944–53	14:1	3·5:1
Weir, 1960[15]	North-East Scotland	1946–56	9:1	1·7:1
MacKay, 1966[16]	West Scotland	1954–63	7:1	1·8:1
	Scotland	1961–63	5·5:1	2·6:1
MacKay (personal communication)	Scotland	1968–70	4·4:1	1·7:1

Changes have occurred earlier and have been well documented in the United Kingdom and elsewhere. Table 2.7 shows that even when using the relatively crude yardstick of ulcer deaths there has been a dramatic change in the gastric ulcer pattern. From a disease

Table 2.5 Ulcer frequency in some different parts of the world.

	Clinical characteristics	Distribution pattern	Reference
Africa	Almost all duodenal, stenosis and obstruction relatively frequent. Almost all men.	Common on W. Coast, Nile/Congo watershed, N. Tanzania, N. Ethiopia. Rare in north savannah of W. Coast, S. Ethiopia, N. Nigeria, most of Zaire and Zambia.	35, 39.
India	Almost all duodenal. Stenosis and obstruction relatively frequent. Almost all men.	Common in south and in Assam; rarer in north.	8, 32–34, 37, 38.
Europe	Duodenal and gastric both generally common (DU two to four times as frequent as GU).	No recognized areas of rarity, but some regional variations, e.g. DU two to three times as frequent in Scotland as in S. England.	13–16, 23–25, 27–31.
N. America	Duodenal ulcer fairly common. Gastric ulcer probably less frequent than in Europe.	Probably fairly even.	12, 22, 26.
Australia	Mainly duodenal ulcer, but relatively high frequency of gastric ulcer in younger women.	Gastric ulcer may be especially common in New South Wales and Queensland.	7, 50–52.

Table 2.7 Proportions of men and women dying with gastric ulcers.

	Perforated ulcer[17]	Ulcer deaths[18]		
	1867	1912	1918	1924
Aged less than 35 years:				
Men	18	182	167	151
Women	96	338	214	109
M:F ratio	0·2:1	0·5:1	0·8:1	1·4:1
Aged 35 years or more:				
Men	42	691	900	1219
Women	43	635	713	620
M:F ratio	1·0:1	1·1:1	1·3:1	2·0:1

predominating in young women in 1867 it has changed in the early part of this century to one which is commoner in men and in the older age groups. The change in the male to female ratio is also illustrated in Table 2.8, which shows the increasing male predominance of peptic ulcer due to the rising frequency of duodenal ulcer in men in Copenhagen.

Table 2.8 Male to female ratio of peptic ulcer in hospital patients in Copenhagen.[19]

	No. of patients	M:F ratio
1901–05	471	0·3:1
1911–15	964	0·9:1
1921–25	1493	1·8:1
1931–35	2559	3·1:1

Analysis of duodenal ulcer frequency patterns has suggested that the disease may have reached a peak prevalence in the mid 1950s and may now be declining in frequency, albeit slowly. Ancillary data which can be adduced to confirm that this decline is probably real can be derived from a fall in diagnoses of duodenal ulcer in York, England and in ulcer perforation in Oxford, England.[25,29] Table 2.9 shows, however, that the decline may be particularly great for gastric ulcer. The reasons for this change are again uncertain. The falling admission ratio cannot be ascribed to the development of new potent methods of treatment, for the decline in ulcer admission rates started prior to the free availability of these treatments in the late 1960s. Perforation is also often the first indication which brings an ulcer to medical attention and the fall in

Table 2.9 Peptic ulcer. Estimated number of in-patients aged 15 years or more from hospital in-patient enquiries in England and Wales, 1959–1974.[23] (Revised and updated).

	Gastric ulcer		Duodenal ulcer	
	Perforated only	Total	Perforated only	Total
1959–62	2567	26 669	5430	38 520
1963–66	1887	21 399	5271	37 948
1967–70	1700	19 560	5259	37 002
1971–74	1478	16 895	4853	33 696
Percentage change first four years to last four years	−42·3	−36·6	−10·6	−12·5

ulcer perforation admissions has been especially marked. In the USA a parallel and perhaps even greater decline in frequency has been noted for both gastric and duodenal ulcer (Table 2.13). A change in the sex ratio of gastric ulcer patients in Eastern Australia has been attributed to a tendency of middle aged women to take aspirin containing compound analgesics, and this is discussed later (p. 27).

Age and sex distribution The frequency of gastric and duodenal ulcer varies with age and in men and women. The overall pattern is not consistent either in time or throughout the world and trends demonstrated in one place may be different in another.

Western Europe and the USA During the last hundred years duodenal ulcer has tended to become predominant with the disease being more common in men than in women, whereas until about 1900 gastric ulcer was the more common, with a greater proportion of women than men.[19–21]

Accurate age-specific incidence rates are difficult to obtain because the diagnosis of ulcer may be established in varying ways. Radiological assessment is reasonably satisfactory for gastric ulcer, though some may be missed, but the same technique will not distinguish between active ulceration and scarring in the duodenal cap, and probably particularly underestimates the frequency of active duodenal ulcer in an undeformed duodenal cap. Table 2.10 shows the incidence rates for gastric and duodenal ulcer in Copenhagen estimated from radiological and operative evidence only.[27,28] It demonstrates that duodenal ulcer is rare before the age of twenty, but that incidence rates then rise progressively into late middle life and old age. By contrast gastric ulcers tend to be less common with incidence rates becoming greater some twenty years later. In general there are greater proportions of men than women

Table 2.10 Gastric and duodenal ulcer in Copenhagen 1963–68.[27,28] Incidence rates per 1000 population (data condensed from published evidence).

Age	Gastric ulcer Men	Gastric ulcer Women	Duodenal ulcer Men	Duodenal ulcer Women
20–	0·1	0·1	0·9	0·2
30–	0·2	0·1	1·3	0·5
40–	0·4	0·3	2·2	1·3
50–	0·7	0·6	3·0	1·4
60–	1·1	0·7	3·2	1·4
70+	1·2	1·0	3·7	2·1

with duodenal ulcer than with gastric ulcer but the difference in sex ratio diminishes in the elderly for gastric ulcer in particular.

The tendency for duodenal ulcer incidence rates to rise progressively with age is new, and Susser[21] has suggested from cohort analyses that a group of people were generally exposed to an environmental influence tending to cause ulcer, but that successive birth cohorts since 1890 had had a diminishing exposure. This hypothesis is compatible with a decreasing frequency of new cases and with a rise in mean patient age, but any basic cause is unknown.

Table 2.11 Ulcer in the United Kingdom and Scandinavia.[27–31] Mean annual incidence rates per 1000 population aged 15 and over.

		Gastric ulcer Men	Gastric ulcer Women	Duodenal ulcer Men	Duodenal ulcer Women
York, England	1952–57[29]	0·5	0·3	2·2	0·6
S.W. Scotland	1957–59[30]	0·4	0·3	5·4	1·3
Rogaland, Norway	1950–52[31]	0·6	0·3	2·4	0·6
Copenhagen County	1963–68[27,28]	0·5	0·4	1·8	0·8

Similar patterns of overall incidence are detectable elsewhere in Europe (Table 2.11). Prevalence rates are much higher, and Table 2.12 shows those found at autopsy in Rotterdam and Leeds. The increase in frequency reflects the fact that prevalence measures overall frequency of active new ulcers as well as old ulcers which may have been present and active long before. In general incidence studies or prevalence studies based primarily on radiological methods, usually without double contrast techniques, must be less

18 *Peptic ulcer*

Table 2.12 Percentage prevalence of gastric and duodenal ulcer according to age and sex in autopsy studies.[1,2]

	Gastric ulcer				Duodenal ulcer			
Age (years)	Leeds		Rotterdam		Leeds		Rotterdam	
	Men	Women	Men	Women	Men	Women	Men	Women
20–	2·7	2·0	0·7	0·4	11·0	3·5	4·9	1·2
30–	4·3	3·0	4·5	1·9	17·0	7·0	8·2	2·5
40–	7·0	3·2	9·8	1·4	16·8	8·0	10·4	5·7
50–	5·6	6·0	9·0	4·4	16·2	5·0	11·5	5·4
60–	4·1	6·0	9·3	6·4	12·0	8·0	10·1	4·6
70+	2·8	6·3	9·7	9·0	10·4	6·0	10·1	6·4

accurate and less sensitive than methods which allow a direct view of the mucosa as by endoscopy as well as post-mortem.

Similar patterns of ulcer frequency with age and sex have been detected in the USA by analyses of spells of incapacity due to ulcer (Table 2.13), and from the results of the National Household Health Survey.[12]

Table 2.13 Age-specific incidence rates of disability due to gastric and duodenal ulcer amongst men, in a manufacturing company. Rates per thousand employees.[26]

Age (years)	Gastric ulcer		Duodenal ulcer	
	1960	1970	1960	1970
20–	1·1	0·1	1·6	0·7
25–	1·1	0·3	4·6	1·3
30–	1·2	0·1	4·5	1·5
35–	1·6	0·7	4·5	2·3
40–	2·1	0·4	5·6	2·7
45–	2·4	0·7	7·4	2·7
50–	3·1	1·2	7·8	3·0
55–	2·7	1·2	6·1	4·9
60–	3·4	1·6	7·5	3·7

India and Africa In general gastric ulcer tends to be rare, and duodenal ulcer much commoner; furthermore, there also tends to be a greater predominance in men.[32-35,39] The data available to support these views is somewhat fragmentary, since comprehensive health care statistics are not available, but Table 2.14 shows the great excess of men over women amongst patients operated upon for ulcer, whether gastric or duodenal, in Madras, India. The same trends can

Table 2.14 Comparison of operative cases of gastric and duodenal ulcer in Madras.[34]

	1942–45	1962–66
Duodenal ulcer:		
Total number	1047	1034
Male:female ratio	26·9:1	13·3:1
Gastric ulcer:		
Total number	66	68
Male:female ratio	22·0:1	9·7:1

be detected in Africa, thus the average male to female ratio found in 18 reported series from high ulcer incidence areas of black Africa[35] was 9·0:1.

The peak age incidence is probably rather lower in both India and Africa than in Western Europe: Tovey and Tunstall found the mean peak age prevalence of active ulcer to be 31 in response to a series of enquiries, ulcer being not uncommon in teenagers and occasionally then associated with pyloric stenosis. The duration of these patterns is uncertain though it seems that gastric and duodenal ulcer were seldom, if ever, reported at necropsy in Africa fifty or more years ago.[35] In India ulcer was probably relatively infrequent fifty years ago, but again the data on which to base an opinion are fragmentary.[36,37] The figures in Table 2.14 show that duodenal ulcer was a common problem in men thirty years ago in Madras, but that duodenal ulcer in women may be becoming a more important disease than previously.[38]

Geographical and environmental factors

Geographical incidence The geographical pattern of ulcer incidence and prevalence has few coherent features. In Europe both duodenal and gastric ulcer are common, with duodenal ulcer being consistently the more frequent by two to threefold (see Tables 2.12 and 2.13). Comparisons between incidence and prevalence figures in different countries are greatly hindered by the lack of uniformity of standards which can be applied in measuring ulcer frequency. Hospital admissions can only account for a minor proportion of all disease and ulcer deaths a much smaller fraction. Perforation can be used as an index of ulcer frequency since it seems that many patients present initially with this complication, but even so the range of figures from which comparisons can be made, and where uniform collection methods have been applied, is limited.

In the United Kingdom the Hospital In-Patient Enquiry (HIPE) collects data on a one-in-ten sample of all hospital admissions and

20 Peptic ulcer

Table 2.15 Regional admission rates of men with duodenal ulcer and gastric ulcer per 1000 population in 1967 in the United Kingdom.[23]

	Duodenal ulcer		Gastric ulcer	
	Perforated only	Total	Perforated only	Total
ENGLAND				
South				
East Anglia	0·07	0·84	0·08	0·54
South West	0·14	0·89	0·02	0·44
Wessex	0·08	0·89	0·08	0·39
Oxford	0·13	0·93	0·04	0·40
North				
Leeds	0·22	1·39	0·07	0·59
Manchester	0·23	1·48	0·10	0·55
Liverpool	0·23	1·59	0·03	0·47
Newcastle	0·31	2·26	0·10	0·59
SCOTLAND	0·45	2·94	0·07	0·57

comparative data are obtainable in different hospital regions; Table 2.15 shows the results obtained in four northerly regions of England and Wales, as well as four southerly regions. There is a clear difference, with duodenal ulcer, either as a group or as perforated ulcer only, being more common in the North than in the South. By contrast, gastric ulcer tends to show no such coherent pattern. This lack of parallelism between gastric and duodenal ulcer admission trends suggests that the figures are more likely to reflect differing disease prevalence than varying management policies in the north and the south. Figures for hospital admissions in Scotland demonstrate the continuity of these differences, with further evidence of increased duodenal ulcer admission rates.[23]

Outside Western Europe the trends again vary. In the United States and Canada duodenal ulcer is probably much commoner than gastric ulcer, the latter disease being much less common than in the United Kingdom. The tendency to regard ulcer as synonymous with a high standard of living in Westernized countries is unjustified. Thus, duodenal ulcer is a common disease in many parts of India and in general there is a contrast between its relative infrequency in the north and frequency in the south. The areas of probable low incidence include parts of Kashmir, Rajasthan and the Punjab, whilst high incidences are found in Kerala, Madras, Mysore, West Bengal, Assam, Bombay and Hyderabad.[32-38] Precise comparisons are hard to make because formal population surveys have been few, and autopsy studies even fewer, but a ten to twentyfold difference in frequency from the common to the rare areas seems likely.

The clinical characteristics of ulcer disease in India outside cities include a very strong predilection for men, a high frequency in young adult life, and a tendency towards pyloric obstruction, with bleeding and perforation being relatively uncommon. The sex ratio has been found to vary from 9:1 to 33:1 with an average of 18:1, a figure which is too high to be readily explained by bias in presentation and diagnosis in men. The tendency for disease to present in young adult life may in part reflect population age distributions and will need confirmation by studies of defined population groups. The relative frequency of pyloric obstruction and infrequency of bleeding and perforation are hard to understand. If late presentation accounted for the rise in the proportions of patients with obstruction then a raised frequency of other complications might reasonably have been expected.

The general distribution of disease conforms to the area where rice is a staple food, whilst it seems to be infrequent in the north where unrefined wheat is the major carbohydrate food. In areas where disease is common this seems to be true for both urban and rural communities, and gastric ulcer is rare.

In Africa the general patterns of incidence are less well defined. The likely areas of high prevalence include the Nile–Congo watershed, Ethiopia and the southern coast of West Africa. Features of the disease are reminiscent of those seen in India. Clinically it tends to be a disease of men, pyloric obstruction is a common feature, gastric ulcer is rare and a rough correlation with the consumption of diets with low residues of unabsorbed carbohydrate is detectable. The general distribution of ulcer disease is shown in Figure 2.1.[35]

Urbanization in East and South Africa seems to be associated with a rising, but still low, overall incidence of duodenal ulcer, and autopsy studies suggest that many of these lesions do not cause significant symptoms and are small and shallow in contrast to the stenosing ulcers seen elsewhere. In the USA there is evidence that ulcer is more prevalent in the black population than in the white, but the difference is not great and may be largely, if not completely, explainable on social class differences.

Socio-economic status and occupation The accepted pattern of ulcer prevalence has been of a disease which increases in frequency from rich to poor for gastric ulcer and from poor to rich for duodenal ulcer. It is now doubtful if this pattern is correct. Table 2.16 shows the mortality rates as standardized mortality ratios for gastric ulcer in the USA and in England and Wales by social class, and with figures for England and Wales in two periods fifty years apart.

Gastric ulcer deaths have been consistently more frequent in

22 *Peptic ulcer*

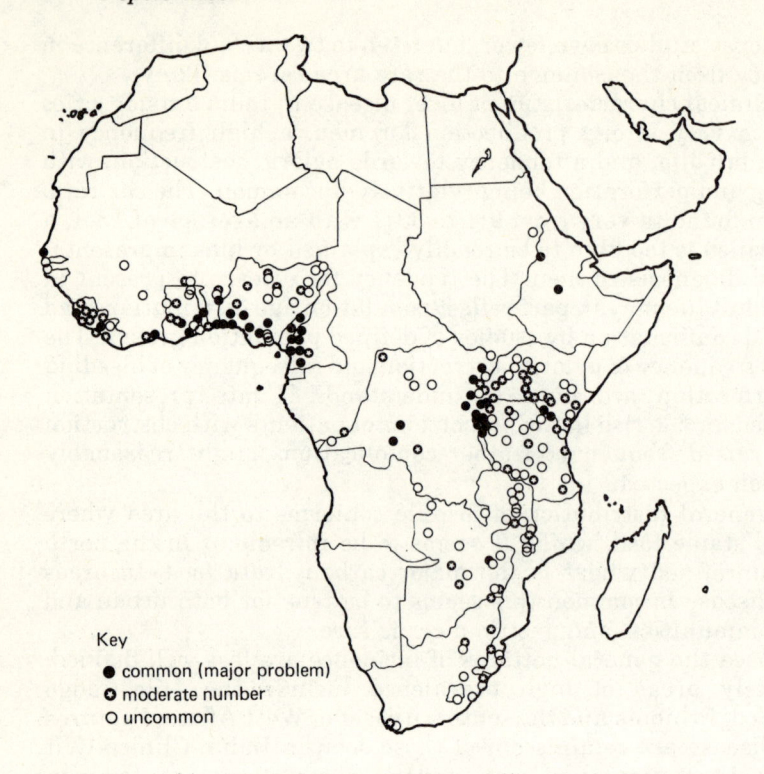

Fig. 2.1 Duodenal ulcer in black populations in Africa south of the Sahara[35]

Key
- ● common (major problem)
- ◉ moderate number
- ○ uncommon

Table 2.16 Ulcer mortality in England and Wales and in the USA in men of differing social class.[5,6] (Standardized mortality ratios).

		Professional and management I	II	Skilled III	Semi-skilled IV	Un-skilled V
England and Wales	Site					
1921–23	Gastric	86		86	105	123
	Duodenal	133		92	92	82
1959–63	Gastric	46	58	94	106	109
	Duodenal	70	84	113	102	136
USA						
1950	Gastric	54	74	94	113	159
	Duodenal	70	84	113	102	136

those in unskilled occupations, and duodenal ulcer deaths now show a similar pattern. Fifty years ago more deaths were recorded than would be expected with duodenal ulcer amongst the relatively affluent in England and Wales despite the fact that they would have been better able to buy a high standard of medical care. Some of the current social class differences may nevertheless be explainable by differences in the quality of medical care obtained by poor and rich people. In the United Kingdom standards of health care are more uniform than in the past, but may still be lower in hospitals in poorer areas, whilst in the USA, health care delivery remains very uneven.

The findings in studies of living patients with ulcer show similar trends to the results of mortality analyses. Table 2.17 shows a

Table 2.17 Observed and expected frequency of gastric and duodenal ulcer in South-West Scotland, 1957 to 1959.[30]

		I	II	III	IV	V
Gastric ulcer	Observed	0	11	12	13	28
	Expected	2	11	30	14	7
Duodenal ulcer	Observed	13	41	125	136	158
	Expected	14	80	218	108	52

higher than expected frequency of duodenal ulcer in those of social class IV or V, as for gastric ulcer. A similar pattern with peptic ulcer (presumably mainly duodenal ulcer) being more frequent in those of lower educational attainment has been detected in the USA and Table 2.18 again illustrates the findings. The table also shows that the association with low educational attainment holds independently of the individuals' smoking habits.

Table 2.18 Educational attainment, smoking habits and ulcer frequency in men and women in Oakland, California.[42]

	Highest educational level attained Percentage with peptic ulcers (age adjusted)		
	Elementary school	High or trade school	College
Men			
Smokers	15·1	13·3	10·7
Non-smokers	7·7	6·2	6·1
Women			
Smokers	9·8	6·8	4·9
Non-smokers	5·0	4·1	3·6

Dietary factors The varying prevalence of ulcer from place to place and from time to time indicates strongly that environmental factors are mainly responsible. These are poorly defined, but there is some limited evidence about possible important factors which has been drawn from broad comparisons of diets in places where ulcer is common and rare, and from surveys conducted in western countries.

In India there is a strong association between the prevalence of ulcer and the consumption of diets of low residue with poor masticatory content, the contrast being between wheat-eating people who make chupatties with unrefined wheat, and those who predominantly eat rice.[36,38,40] If a diet of high residue or masticatory content prevent ulcer the reasons are unclear. Such a diet has no specific neutralizing characteristics, nor is there any reason to believe that it is less of a stimulus to gastric acid output than a low residue diet. The suggestion that a large volume of saliva produced in chewing diet of high residue will buffer gastric contents is unconvincing, since the buffering capacity of saliva is low.

An alternative suggestion has been that liability to ulcer can be associated with food additives such as spices and chillies. However, the use of such food additives seemed to be similar in both North and South India. Some limited epidemiological evidence suggests that the consumption of fresh vegetables may protect against ulcer, but the mechanism is unclear.[38]

A correlation between low residue African diets and liability to duodenal ulcer can also be detected; thus the diet on the south coast of West Africa where ulcer is common contains a high proportion of carbohydrate as tubers with a low fibrous residue.[35]

Knowledge of potentially important characteristics of western diets is even more inadequate. There are no communities with clearly distinct diets, and the high mobility of western populations, together with their changing dietary habits, makes studies difficult.

Questionnaires administered to university students at Harvard and Pennsylvania in the 1930s were recently followed up and the occurrence of ulcer, mainly as duodenal ulcer, was correlated with the answers obtained well before the ulcers were diagnosed or caused symptoms.[41] Those students who took more coffee, or soft drinks of the cola variety subsequently had a higher incidence of ulcer. By contrast, tea and alcohol consumption could not be correlated with later occurrence of ulcer; whilst those who drank milk tended to be relatively protected (Table 2.19).

The associations of ulcer with coffee and soft drink intake, and the apparent protective effect of milk were detectable independently when paired analyses were made to allow for complicating variables. The meaning of these associations is unclear; direct causal relationships should not necessarily be assumed since each of the beverages could be acting as a marker for other substances not included in the survey.

Table 2.19 Age- and interval-adjusted incidence rates of peptic ulcer per 1000 respondents in former students at Harvard and Pennsylvania Universities in relation to their beverage consumption habits.[41]

Beverage		Incidence rate
Coffee (cups daily)	2+	31·7
	1	24·5
	Nil	17·7
Tea	Yes	20·9
	No	21·3
Soft drinks	Yes	22·0
	No	14·9
Alcohol	Yes	9·9
	No	10·6
Milk (glasses daily)	4+	18·6
	1–3	15·4
	Nil	30·3

Other evidence[42] obtained by retrospective case control questionnaire has suggested that alcohol consumption was not associated with liability to ulcer but the same study also failed to show any association with coffee consumption possibly for methodological reasons.[43] Given the known failings of retrospective questionnaire analyses, these results must be given less weight than the prospective inquiries of Paffenbarger and his colleagues.

Other factors

Smoking Death rates with peptic ulcer are higher in smokers than in non-smokers,[44,45] and ulcer itself is found more often in smokers than in non-smokers. However, these findings do not necessarily imply that smoking is an important causal factor in peptic ulceration. Increased death rates in individuals with peptic ulceration could be attributed at least in part, for instance, to deaths following surgery for ulcer which were primarily due to postoperative respiratory complications. Likewise, an increased frequency of smokers amongst those with ulcers compared with control individuals[46] could be due in part to a common social class pattern for peptic ulceration and smoking if control people were not similarly matched for social class.

Examination of the smoking habits of Massachusetts physicians[47] showed that those with gastric or duodenal ulcers had smoked more than those who did not have ulcers, and those with duodenal ulcers had started smoking at an earlier age (Table 2.20). However, when

26 *Peptic ulcer*

Table 2.20 Past smoking habits of Massachusetts physicians.[47]

Age	Percentage smoking cigarettes at set ages		
	Duodenal ulcer	Gastric ulcer	Control individuals
20	52·7	40·1	38·9
30	65·0	76·9	53·7

smokers only were considered the patients and controls were similar in the number of years for which they had smoked, the amount smoked per day and in the proportion who had ultimately stopped, suggesting that liability to ulcer and to smoke were separately derived from some other cause.

Further evidence to support the suggestion that smoking may be a causal factor of peptic ulceration comes from the data of Paffenbarger and his colleagues,[41] who compared the smoking habits found in college students with their later histories of ulcer (Table 2.21). Smoking was more prevalent in those who developed ulcers

Table 2.21 Smoking habits prior to development of ulcer in American college students.[41]

	Number of respondents	Number of ulcer patients	Age- and interval-adjusted incidence rates per 1000
Smokers	9 061	184	21·1
Non-smokers	14 702	229	15·2

later, though the association was weaker than those detected in the same students with coffee or with soft drinks consumption.

Taken overall, the association between smoking and ulcer is weak, and the habit can at best play only a minor causal role in ulcer development.

Alcohol It is commonly supposed that alcohol consumption both causes peptic ulceration and exacerbates its symptoms. The evidence in support of either concept is weak. Paffenbarger and his colleagues in their inquiry into the habits of American college students[41] found no association between alcohol intake as a student and later liability to ulcer, nor was any association detected in a population survey in California.[42] A high proportion of cirrhotic patients have been found to have ulcers,[48] and this could theoretically be due to a common association with alcohol consumption.

Peptic ulcer 27

However, there is no evidence to show that peptic ulceration is a particular problem in the cirrhotic alcoholic, and one study suggested that ulcer was, if anything, more common in cryptogenic cirrhosis than in alcoholic cirrhosis.[49]

Current evidence suggests that mild to moderate alcohol consumption may have little or no effect on liability to ulcer, whilst the effects of heavy consumption are unclear.

Aspirin Two distinct problems need examination, firstly the liability of aspirin to induce chronic peptic ulceration, and secondly, the liability of aspirin to cause acute upper gastrointestinal bleeding. The tendency for gastric ulcer and gastric ulcer complications to become more frequent in middle-aged women in Australia (Table 2.22)[50–52] has been attributed to the habitual intake of compound

Table 2.22 Male to female ratio of gastric ulcer patients admitted to hospitals in Sydney, New South Wales.[50,51]

	Number of patients	Male to female ratio
1930–39	427	2·5:1
1946–55	1388	1·3:1
1959–61	963	0·8:1

analgesics containing aspirin, and case-control comparisons have substantiated the association. The general extent of the risk is uncertain, but it seems likely that this form of drug abuse can account for only a minor proportion of all gastric ulcer detected.

The association has been found in North America, notably in the Boston Collaborative Drug Enquiry;[53] the evidence there (Table 2.23) suggests only a very limited risk in those defined as heavy consumers and no risk in light or occasional takers of aspirin. Overall the risk in heavy consumers was calculated to be of the order of 10 per 100 000 per year.

Table 2.23 Habitual aspirin intake greater than three times a week for three months in patients with acute gastrointestinal bleeding and with chronic gastric ulcer in Boston, USA.[53]

	Total number of cases	Aspirin users	Standardized morbidity ratio
Acute upper gastro-intestinal bleeding	88	14 (15·9%)	2·1
Chronic gastric ulcer	29	5 (19·2%)	3·4
Controls	14 813	1015 (6·9%)	—

By contrast, the liability of aspirin to cause acute upper gastrointestinal bleeding has been suggested in a number of case control comparisons between recent aspirin intake in patients with bleeding and in matched controls. The association has been most obvious in those with normal barium meals and who have therefore been assumed to have acute gastric erosions (Table 2.24). A simple

Table 2.24 Percentage of recent aspirin takers in patients with haematemesis or melaena and in control individuals.

	X-ray negative	Ulcer Duodenal	Gastric	Control
London[54]	60	44	33	17[a]
London[55]	65	52	49	32[b]
Glasgow[56]	62	39	47	5[c]
Sheffield[57]	70	49		44[d]

a Dyspeptic outpatients
b All other in-patients
c Control in right hand bed of patient
d Accident and emergency cases

deduction from the differences found is that aspirin is a clear and important cause of acute upper gastrointestinal bleeding; however, there are reasons why this interpretation may be inadequate.[58] It is not possible to determine whether any aspirin intake in the bleeding group was the cause of the bleeding or consequential upon symptoms either of the bleeding itself (for instance, faintness misinterpreted before overt haemorrhage as influenza), or of the lesion causing that bleeding. Secondly, the control groups used have not been drawn from the general population, hospital in-patients and out-patients are not necessarily representative, and have not always been properly matched, since analgesic intake for minor ailments can vary with age, sex and probably social class. Analgesic intake is common in the general population and at least one-third of a population sample have been found to admit to recent intake before questioning. Thirdly, in no published study has paracetamol (acetaminophen) intake been used as a positive control to examine for systematic bias in drug consumption. Our own data suggest that recent paracetamol intake is detectable twice as frequently in bleeding patients as in a random population control, suggesting that systematic bias may indeed be important. Fourthly, re-exposure to aspirin in aspirin bleeders does not precipitate acute haemorrhage, but only micro-bleeding as in normal individuals. It has therefore been suggested that the coincidence of aspirin intake with a second factor, such as alcohol consumption, may be necessary, but again, the evidence does not withstand examination. In general terms the proportion of alcohol takers has been found to be no different in those with aspirin associated bleeding than in those who had not taken aspirin, except in one study where a modest association with duodenal ulcer (but not with gastritis) was detected (Table 2.25).

Table 2.25 Observed and expected numbers of coincident takers of aspirin and alcohol in Aberdeen, Scotland in patients with haematemesis and melaena[59] (adapted).*

Diagnosis		Takers of aspirin and alcohol together	
		Observed	Expected by chance
Duodenal ulcer	M	22	13
	F	4	2
Gastric ulcer	M	3	2
	F	3	1
Gastritis	M	8	11
	F	1	2

Taken overall it seems likely that aspirin intake is, at most, a minor cause of acute upper gastrointestinal bleeding, and this point is exemplified by the Boston Collaborative Study,[53] where no risk of bleeding was detectable in light consumers of aspirin, but that an approximate doubling of risk of 15 per 100 000 per year was estimated to occur in heavy takers (defined as those taking four or more doses a week for at least the previous three months).

Non-steroidal antirheumatoid drugs These are widely reputed to exacerbate dyspepsia, to cause ulceration and to induce bleeding. All these opinions may be well based and there is experimental evidence to suggest that these drugs may have harmful effects on the stomach, but no epidemiological comparisons of ulcer or complication frequency in patients taking and not taking antirheumatoid drugs exist. The suggestion that greater curve gastric ulceration is a specific complication of antirheumatoid therapy is ill-founded.

Corticosteroid drugs Adrenocorticosteroid therapy has been generally believed to cause the development or activation of peptic ulcers. A review of ulcer frequency in 42 controlled studies of corticosteroid therapy for a variety of diseases suggested that treatment was unassociated with peptic ulcer.[60] The conclusion may be open to question: there were a total of 38 ulcers in 2985 patients receiving corticosteroids compared with 18 in 2346 controls, a

* Figures recalculated for analysis by individual diagnostic category.

relative risk of 1·66. This would suggest that ulcer is indeed a potential complication of corticosteroid therapy, but 32 of the total of 56 ulcers developed in one trial in patients with cirrhosis. In the remaining patients the frequency of ulcer was 17 in 2816 (0·6%) compared with 7 in 2181 (0·3%) in the steroid and control groups respectively; the difference is perceptible but the overall frequency so low that for all practical purposes any risk of ulcer development due to steroid therapy can be regarded as unimportant.

Associated diseases

A wide variety of other diseases have been reported to be associated with gastric or duodenal ulceration, but close examination of the supporting data suggests that many of those claims are insecurely founded.[61] Three important causes of interpretative difficulty can be identified.

First, any group of patients with a chronic disease who are followed clinically for a lengthy period of time will be likely to have a second disease found simply because close scrutiny will tend to identify abnormalities which could well have remained unknown in the ordinary population. An example of the likely effects of close follow-up is given in Table 2.26. Two groups of patients with liver

Table 2.26 Overall frequency of ulcer in patients with liver disease in the USA.[48]

	Total number of patients	Ulcer percentage Pre-inclusion assessment	Post-inclusion follow up
Control	265	11·7	8·7
Shunt	245	7·7	11·8

disease and oesophageal varices were randomly allocated to treatment by portocaval shunt or by simple medical management. Approximately one in ten of the patients were known to have ulcers beforehand, and one in ten were found to have ulcers during the follow-up period in both operative and non-operative groups.[48]

Second, groups of patients with disease may have a second disease identified by two means, either those with disease A may incidentally be found to have disease B, or else those with disease A may incidentally be identified after referral with disease B. The combination of these effects could lead to an artificial apparent association. Thus, Fig. 2.2 shows that if the overall frequency of peptic ulcer in a population is one in ten, whether patients are otherwise

Peptic ulcer 31

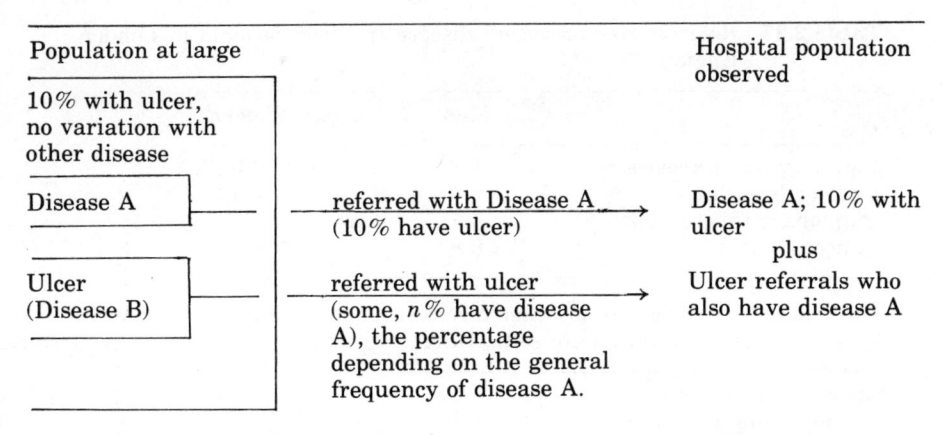

Population at large		Hospital population observed
10% with ulcer, no variation with other disease		
Disease A	referred with Disease A (10% have ulcer) →	Disease A; 10% with ulcer
		plus
Ulcer (Disease B)	referred with ulcer (some, n% have disease A), the percentage depending on the general frequency of disease A. →	Ulcer referrals who also have disease A

∴ The observed hospital frequency of ulcer with disease A reflects the sum of the cases of disease A + ulcer arriving by each referral route. If ulcer is a common route of referral and disease A is often detected secondarily in this group, then the observed hospital frequency of ulcer plus disease A will appear very inflated.

Fig. 2.2 Effect of a varying referral rate for a second, non-ulcer disease on the apparent association between ulcer and that second disease[62] (Adapted)

healthy or whether they have another disease then the apparent frequency of ulcer in the population referred to hospital is in part determined by the referral rates for the associated disease. If an 'associated' disease has a particularly high referral rate the large number of referrals with that disease will minimize the effects of the alternative route of referral because of ulcer. If the second disease has a low rate of referral then the alternative route of referral primarily because of ulcer, but with the second disease, will cause an apparent association of ulcer with the second disease.[62]

A third means of apparent association arises through a common tendency for ulcer and a second disease to occur in the same group of people, common social class or common age group or the same sex, where the ulcer and the second disease are not in fact associated at all.

When all these points are borne in mind the likelihood that most apparent associations between ulcer and a second disease are in fact true becomes very small.

The relative risks of particular second diseases being found in patients with duodenal ulcer are shown in Tables 2.27[63] and 2.28.[64] In neither of these studies is it possible to judge whether the generally increased rates of disease incidence reflect selection bias or a true change. The findings in the general practice survey in the United Kingdom may in part be due to selection for a common social

Table 2.27 Relative risk of second disease in ulcer patients in London, England.[63]

	Men	Women
Coronary heart disease	1·8	2·0
Chronic bronchitis	2·0	2·4
Pulmonary tuberculosis	5·1	4·0
Cancer	0·8	1·1

Table 2.28 Relative risk of other diseases in physicians with duodenal ulcer in Massachusetts, USA.[64]

Myocardial Infarction	1·7
Chronic lung disease	2·3
Rheumatoid arthritis	1·6
Diabetes mellitus	1·0

class. The findings in the American physician study of a relative risk of unity in diabetics for duodenal ulcer suggests a tendency to exaggerated ratios, perhaps from overreporting with a second chronic disease, because other evidence suggests that diabetics are likely to have a diminished risk of duodenal ulcer compared with the general population,[65] probably due to their increased frequency of atrophic gastritis and to the occurrence of autovagotomy which seems to be relatively common in diabetics.[66]

Cardiovascular disease Suggested specific associations include those between duodenal ulcer and aortic aneurysm,[67] and gastric ulcer and aortic calcification.[68] However, control matching was not wholly adequate in these studies and therefore the significance of the findings is doubtful. Two population studies with controls have suggested an association between lower blood pressure and liability to ulcer, and these are difficult to reconcile with other suggestions of association with degenerative vascular disease.[41,69]

Respiratory disease Chronic lung disease has been associated with peptic ulcer by some,[2,63] but denied by others.[70] The overall frequency of ulcer in patients with chronic lung disease, who are usually men of low social class, does not however appear especially high (just under 18% in one study)[2] when possible biasing factors are taken into account, as well as the high general population frequency of ulcer.

Renal disease A high frequency of duodenal ulcer has been found in patients with chronic renal failure undergoing maintenance dialysis or after transplantation.[71,72] Although acid output in uraemic patients has been found to be normal or low, patients receiving haemodialysis tend to have hypergastrinaemia and high acid outputs.[71] Corticosteroid therapy may predispose to ulcer in transplant patients, though supporting evidence that these drugs will induce ulcer is questionable.[60]

Endocrine abnormalities Postulated associations with adrenocortical hyperplasia or adenomata are poorly supported by facts. Hyperparathyroid patients are also commonly supposed to be prone to ulcer, but the overall frequency of 14% found in ten collected series is scarcely outside the general prevalence of peptic ulcer, active and inactive, in the community.[73]

Joint disease Surveys of ulcer frequency in patients with joint disease have been mainly devoted to trying to determine if treatment affects ulcer frequency. Conclusions have been inconsistent, and ulcer frequency taken overall does not seem high.[61]

Gastrointestinal disease The high frequency of ulcer detected in cirrhotics[48] may reflect a true increase, a common response to alcohol (though the role of alcohol in inducing peptic ulceration here, or in inducing ulcer complications is doubtful), or simply the effects of continued interest and investigation during follow-up (see Table 2.26 and p. 31). Gastric hypersecretion appears to be inducible by small bowel resection,[74] but there is no compelling evidence that ulcer is particularly frequent in patients with Crohn's disease, resected or unresected.

The association of severe ulceration with gastrin hypersecretion in the Zollinger–Ellison syndrome is well known, but the role of more prosaic abnormalities such as atrophic gastritis in affecting ulcer frequency is unclear. In a single survey of 116 patients with biopsy proven atrophic gastritis, two gastric ulcers were found 19 to 23 years later, a finding which is likely to differ by little from population expectation.[75]

Genetic factors

Peptic ulceration occurs commonly within families, but since the disease itself is frequent this aggregation could simply be a chance phenomenon. Evidence that familial aggregation results from an inherited liability to peptic ulcer arises from several sources.

Family studies Doll and Kellock[76] showed in 1951 that peptic ulcer occurred rather over twice as frequently in the brothers and sisters of patients as in the general population. Furthermore, they found that the relatives of patients with gastric or with duodenal ulcers

34 Peptic ulcer

tended to develop the same sort of ulcers, and that liability to ulcer tends to be the same in different generations as well as in the same generation.

Genetic markers   There is ample evidence that individuals of blood group O have an increased liability to ulcer,[77,78] this being particularly strong for duodenal ulcer and for ulcer associated with bleeding. In addition, those people who are non-secretors and are therefore genetically incapable of producing their ABO(H) blood group substances in their mucous secretions (these are replaced by Lewis substances) are also more liable to ulcer (and probably operation for ulcer but not to acute bleeding),[79] this characteristic being inherited independently of the ABO blood groups (Tables 2.29–2.31).[79,81] The

Table 2.29 ABO blood groups in gastric and duodenal ulcer patients and controls.[78]

	Percentage having blood group				Total number
	O	A	B	AB	
Gastric	52·4	38·1	7·7	1·8	599
Duodenal	56·5	32·9	7·8	2·7	946
Control	45·8	42·2	8·9	3·1	10 000

Table 2.30 Percentage of group O in duodenal ulcer patients with symptoms of pain or obstruction and bleeding.[79]

	Number of patients with group O	Percentage of patients with group O	Total number
Pain or obstruction only	408	52·3	780
Haematemesis or melaena	323	59·3	545

Table 2.31 Percentage of non-secretors in duodenal and gastric ulcer patients and in control individuals.[80]

	Number of non-secretors	Percentage of non-secretors	Total number
Gastric	116	28·7	404
Duodenal	543	35·3	1540
Control	590	24·2	2435

basis for these associations is unclear and no consistent evidence is available to link them with any specific patterns of acid secretory or pepsinogen output. A contrast can be drawn with gastric cancer or pernicious anaemia, weakly associated with blood group A, but not with ABO(H) non-secretion, but again the cause of these associations is not understood.

Serum pepsinogen Pepsinogens are separable electrophoretically and by radio-immunoassay into two or more components. Recently a higher proportion of individuals with gastric or duodenal ulcer have been found to produce higher serum levels of group I pepsinogen identified by radio-immunoassay than control individuals, the results giving a bimodal distribution.[82] Further evidence is needed to determine whether this difference is genetically determined and affects liability to ulcer disease.

Recently an association has been suggested between liability to ulcer and HLA B-5.[83] This association which is stronger than that for the ABO blood groups or secretor status (relative liability in HLA B-5 versus the remainder 2·9:1) needs confirmation.*

Psychological factors

Psychological factors are commonly considered to be important in the genesis or exacerbation of ulcer, but supporting data are poor, for little information collected has been collected prior to ulcer development, and data collected later must be of doubtful validity due to the effect of the disease upon recall of events. Examination of Harvard students suggested that those who lately developed ulcers were no more prone to anxiety than their peers.[41] However, students who died in whom ulcer was considered a primary or subsidiary cause of death were more likely to have had symptoms such as palpitations and sleeplessness as students, in addition the chances of early paternal death were greater than in controls.[84]

An asthenic body form has also been considered by some to be associated with liability to ulcer, but no difference has been found in this respect between those who later developed ulcers and control individuals.

References

1. Watkinson, G. (1960). The incidence of chronic peptic ulcer found at necropsy. *Gut* **1**, 14–31.
2. Levij, I. S., De la Fuente, A. A. (1963). A post mortem study of gastric and duodenal peptic lesions. *Gut* **4**, 349–59.
3. *Registrar General's Statistical Review for 1967.* (1968). London, HMSO.
4. *Registrar General's Statistical Review for 1968.* (1970). London, HMSO.
5. Guralnick, L. (1963). Mortality by occupational level and cause of death

* Not confirmed in later studies.

among men 20 to 60 years of age. *United States Vital Statistics Special Reports*, **53**, 439.
6. *Registrar General's Decennial Supplements: Occupational Mortality Tables for 1921–23, 1949–53, 1959–63.* (1927), (1958), (1971). London, HMSO.
7. Gillies, M. A., Skyring, A. (1969). Gastric and duodenal ulcer. The association between aspirin ingestion, smoking and family history of ulcer. *Medical Journal of Australia*, **2**, 280–5.
8. Malhotra, S. L., Majumdar, C. T., Bardoloi, P. C. (1964). Peptic ulcer in Assam. *Gut* **5**, 355–8.
9. Medalie, J. H., Birnbaum, D., Goldbourt, U., Neufeld, H. N., Riss, E., Oron, D., Perlstein, T. (1972). Peptic ulcer history among 10 000 adult males. I, Prevalence and Incidence. *Israel Journal of Medical Science* **8**, 1673–9.
10. Doll, R., Avery Jones, F., Bukatsch, M. M. (1946). *Occupational Factors in the Aetiology of Gastric and Duodenal Ulcers with an Estimate of their Incidence in the General Population.* Medical Research Council Special Report Series No. 276. London, HMSO.
11. Weir, R. D., Backett, E. M. (1968). Studies of the epidemiology of peptic ulcer in a rural community: Prevalence and natural history of dyspepsia and peptic ulcer. *Gut* **9**, 75–83.
12. Mendeloff, A. I., Dunn, J. P. (1971). *Digestive Diseases. Vital and Health Statistics Monographs.* American Public Health Association. Cambridge, Mass., Harvard University Press.
13. Illingworth, C. F. W., Scott, L. D. W., Jamieson, R. A. (1944). Acute perforated peptic ulcer. Frequency and incidence in the West of Scotland. *British Medical Journal* **2**, 617–20; 655–8.
14. Jamieson, R. A. (1955). Acute perforated peptic ulcer. Frequency and incidence in the West of Scotland. *British Medical Journal* **2**, 222–7.
15. Weir, R. D. (1960). Perforated peptic ulcer in North-East Scotland. *Scottish Medical Journal* **5**, 257–64.
16. Mackay, C. (1966). Perforated peptic ulcer in the West of Scotland; a survey of 5343 cases during 1954–62. *British Medical Journal* **1**, 701–5.
17. Brinton, W. (1867). *On the Pathology, Symptoms and Treatment of Ulcer of the Stomach.* London, Churchill.
18. *Registrar General's Statistical Reviews for 1912, 1918, 1924.* (1914), (1920), (1925). London, HMSO.
19. Hansen, J. L. (1937). Investigation on frequency of peptic ulcer with special regard to distribution between two sexes. *Ugeskrift für Laeger* **99**, 1145–51.
20. Jennings, D. (1940). Perforated peptic ulcer. Changes in age-incidence and sex-distribution in the last 150 years. *Lancet* **1**, 395–8; 444–7.
21. Susser, M. (1967). Causes of peptic ulcer: a selective epidemiologic review. *Journal of Chronic Diseases* **20**, 435–56.
22. Mendeloff, A. I. (1974). What has been happening to duodenal ulcer? *Gastroenterology* **67**, 1020–2.
23. Brown, R. C., Langman, M. J. S., Lambert, P. M. (1976). Hospital admissions for peptic ulcer during 1958–72. *British Medical Journal* **1**, 35–7.
24. Pulvertaft, C. N. (1968). Comments on the incidence and natural history of gastric and duodenal ulcer. *Postgraduate Medical Journal* **44**, 597–602.

25. Sanders, R. (1967). Incidence of perforated duodenal and gastric ulcer in Oxford. *Gut* **8**, 58–63.
26. Almy, T. P. (1975). Prevalence and significance of digestive disease. *Gastroenterology* **68**, 1351–71.
27. Bonnevie, O. (1975). The incidence of gastric ulcer in Copenhagen County. *Scandinavian Journal of Gastroenterology* **10**, 231–9.
28. Bonnevie, O. (1975). The incidence of duodenal ulcer in Copenhagen County. *Scandinavian Journal of Gastroenterology* **10**, 385–93.
29. Pulvertaft, C. N. (1959). Peptic ulcer in town and country. *British Journal of Social and Preventive Medicine* **13**, 131–8.
30. Litton, A., Murdoch, W. R. (1963). Peptic ulcer in South-West Scotland. *Gut* **4**, 360–6.
31. Sponheim, N. (1960). Incidence and prevalence of peptic ulcer in a part of the country. *Nordisk Medicin* **63**, 377–85.
32. Malhotra, S. L. (1964). Peptic ulcer in India and its aetiology. *Gut* **5**, 412–16.
33. Malhotra, S. L. (1967). Epidemiological study of peptic ulcer in the South of India and the ulcer change. *Gut* **8**, 180–8.
34. Madanagopalan, N., Subramanian, R., Krishnan, M. N. (1968). Comparative study of operated cases of peptic ulcer in Madras in the 1940s and 1960s. *Gut* **9**, 69–74.
35. Tovey, F. I., Tunstall, M. (1975). Duodenal ulcer in black populations in Africa South of the Sahara. *Gut* **16**, 564–76.
36. Cleave, T. L. (1962). *Peptic ulcer*. Bristol, J. Wright.
37. Dogra, J. R. (1940). Studies on peptic ulcer in S. India. *Indian Journal of Medical Research* **28**, 145–61.
38. Tovey, F. I. (1972). Duodenal ulcer in Mysone. *Tropical and Geographical Medicine* **24**, 107–17.
39. Konstam, P. (1954). Peptic ulceration in Southern Nigeria. *Lancet* **2**, 1039–40.
40. Malhotra, S. L. (1964). Peptic ulcer in India and its aetiology. *Gut* **5**, 412–16.
41. Paffenbarger, R. S., Wing, A. L., Hyde, R. T. (1974). Chronic disease in former college students. *American Journal of Epidemiology* **100**, 307–15.
42. Freidman, G. D., Siegelaub, A. B., Seltzer, C. C. (1974). Cigarettes, alcohol, coffee and peptic ulcer. *New England Journal of Medicine* **290**, 469–73.
43. Paffenbarger, R. S., Wing, A. L., Hyde, R. T. (1974). Coffee, cigarettes and peptic ulcer. *New England Journal of Medicine* **290**, 1091.
44. Doll, R., Hill, A. B. (1964). Mortality in relation to smoking: 10 years observation of British doctors. *British Medical Journal* **1**, 1399–1410; 1460–7.
45. Hammond, E. C., Horn, D. (1958). Smoking and death rates – report of forty-four months of follow-up of 187 783 men; I. *Journal of the American Medical Association* **166**, 1294–1308.
46. Trowell, O. A. (1934). The relation of tobacco smoking to the incidence of chronic duodenal ulcer. *Lancet* **1**, 808–9.
47. Monson, R. R. (1970). Cigarette smoking and body form in peptic ulcer. *Gastroenterology* **58**, 337–44.
48. Phillips, M. M., Ramsby, G. R., Conn, H. O. (1975). Portocaval anastomosis and peptic ulcer: a non-association. *Gastroenterology* **68**,

121-31.
49. Tabaqchali, S., Dawson, A. M. (1964). Peptic ulcer and gastric secretion in patients with liver disease. *Gut* **5**, 417-21.
50. Billington, B. P. (1963). The Australian gastric ulcer change: interstate variations. *Australasian Annals of Medicine* **12**, 153-9.
51. Billington, B. P. (1965). Observations from New South Wales on the changing incidence of gastric ulcer in Australia. *Gut* **6**, 121-33.
52. Gillies, M. A., Skyring, A. (1969). Gastric and duodenal ulcer. The association between aspirin ingestion, smoking and family history of ulcer. *Medical Journal of Australia* **2**, 280-5.
53. Levy, M. (1974). Aspirin use in patients with major upper gastrointestinal bleeding and peptic ulcer disease. *New England Journal of Medicine* **290**, 1158-62.
54. Alvarez, A. S., Summerskill, W. H. J. (1958). Gastrointestinal haemorrhage and salicylates. *Lancet* **2**, 920-5.
55. Valman, H. B., Parry, D. J., Coghill, N. F. (1968). Lesions associated with gastroduodenal haemorrhage in relation to aspirin intake. *British Medical Journal* **4**, 661-3.
56. Muir, A., Cossar, I. A. (1955). Aspirin and ulcer. *British Medical Journal* **2**, 7-12.
57. Allibone, A., Flint, F. J. (1958). Gastrointestinal haemorrhage and salicylates. *Lancet* **2**, 1121.
58. Langman, M. J. S. (1970). Epidemiological evidence for the association of aspirin and acute gastrointestinal bleeding. *Gut* **11**, 627-34.
59. Needham, C. D., Kyle, J., Jones, P. F., Johnston, S. J., Kerridge, D. F. (1971). Aspirin and alcohol in gastrointestinal haemorrhage. *Gut* **12**, 819-21.
60. Conn, H. O., Blitzer, B. L. (1976). Non-association of adrenocorticosteroid therapy and peptic ulcer. *New England Journal of Medicine* **294**, 473-9.
61. Langman, M. J. S., Cooke, A. R. (1976). Gastric and duodenal ulcer and their associated diseases. *Lancet* **1**, 680-3.
62. Donaldson, R. M. (1975). Factors complicating observed associations between peptic ulcer and other diseases. *Gastroenterology* **68**, 1608-14.
63. Fry, J. (1964). Peptic ulcer: a profile. *British Medical Journal* **2**, 809-12.
64. Monson, R. R. (1970). Duodenal ulcer as a second disease. *Gastroenterology* **59**, 712-16.
65. Dotevall, G. (1959). Incidence of peptic ulcer in diabetes mellitus. *Acta medica Scandinavica* **164**, 463-77.
66. Hosking, D. J., Moody, F., Stewart, I. M., Atkinson, M. (1975). Vagal impairment of gastric secretion in diabetic autonomic neuropathy. *British Medical Journal* **2**, 588-90.
67. Jones, A. W., Kirk, R. S., Bloor, K. (1970). The association between aneurysm of the abdominal aorta and peptic ulceration. *Gut* **11**, 679-84.
68. Elkeles, A. W. (1964). Gastric ulcer in the aged and calcified atherosclerosis. *American Journal of Roentgenology* **91**, 744-50.
69. Medalie, J. H., Neufeld, H. N., Goldbourt, U., Kahn, H. A., Riss, E., Oron, D. (1970). Association between blood pressure and peptic ulcer incidence. *Lancet* **2**, 1225-6.
70. Allibone, A., Flint, F. J. (1958). Bronchitis, aspirin, smoking, and other factors in the aetiology of peptic ulcer. *Lancet* **2**, 179-82.
71. Shepherd, A. M. M., Stewart, W. K., Wormsley, K. G. (1973). Peptic

ulceration in chronic renal failure. *Lancet* **1**, 1357–9.
72. Hadjiyannakis, E. J., Evans, J. B., Smellie, W. A. B., Calne, R. Y. (1971). Gastrointestinal complications after renal transplantation. *Lancet* **2**, 781–5.
73. Barreras, R. F. (1973). Calcium and gastric secretion. *Gastroenterology* **64**, 1168–84.
74. Buxton, B. (1974). Small bowel resection and gastric acid hypersecretion. *Gut* **15**, 229–38.
75. Siurala, M., Lehtola, J., Ihamaki, T. (1974). Atrophic gastritis and its sequelae. *Scandinavian Journal of Gastroenterology* **9**, 441–6.
76. Doll, R., Kellock, T. D. (1951). The separate inheritance of gastric and duodenal ulcers. *Annals of Eugenics* **16**, 231–40.
77. Langman, M. J. S. (1973). Blood groups and alimentary disorders. *Clinics in Gastroenterology* **2**, 497–506.
78. Aird, I., Bentall, H. H., Mehigan, J. A., Roberts, J. A. F. (1954). The blood groups in relation to peptic ulceration and carcinoma of colon, rectum, breast and bronchus. *British Medical Journal* **2**, 315–21.
79. Langman, M. J. S., Doll, R. (1965). ABO blood groups and secretor status in relation to clinical characteristics of peptic ulcer. *Gut* **6**, 270–3.
80. Clarke, C. A., Edwards, J. W., Haddock, D. R. W., Howel Evans, A. W., McConnell, R. B., Sheppard, P. M. (1956). ABO blood groups and secretor character in duodenal ulcer. *British Medical Journal* **2**, 725–31.
81. McConnell, R. B. (1966). *The Genetics of Gastrointestinal Disorders*. London, Oxford University Press.
82. Samloff, I. M., Liebman, W. M., Panitch, N. M. (1975). Serum group I pepsinogens by radio-immunoassay in control subjects and patients with peptic ulcer. *Gastroenterology* **69**, 83–90.
83. Rotter, J. I., Rimoin, D. L., Gursky, J. M., Terasaki, P., Sturdevant, R. A. L. (1977). HLA-B5 associated with duodenal ulcer. *Gastroenterology* **73**, 438–40.
84. Polednak, A. P. (1974). Some early characteristics of peptic ulcer decedents. *Gastroenterology* **67**, 1094–100.

3
Gastrointestinal cancer

Though data are incomplete, examination of the available incidence and mortality figures throughout the world shows that the frequency of gastrointestinal cancer varies very greatly. These fluctuations are, in general, far too large to be explainable by anomalies of reporting systems or by differences in the age structures of the populations under review.

Certain general features can be discerned in the figures. Geographical fluctuations can usually be detected as smooth and gradual trends from one area to another, for instance in the diminishing frequency of gastric cancer from Eastern to Western Europe. Abrupt transitions do occasionally occur, as evidenced by the widely varying frequency of oesophageal cancer on the south side of the Caspian Sea.

Specific types of cancer have separate incidence patterns, thus, gastric and oesophageal cancer have different areas of high and low frequency, but occasionally associated variations can be distinguished. Thus, colonic and rectal cancer tend to be of high or of low frequency in the same area, and inverse correlations can be found, notably in the frequency of gastric and colonic cancer.

Temporal changes in incidence can also be recognized, with, for instance, a falling frequency of gastric cancer in the USA. Sometimes such trends may be due to improving diagnostic precision, for instance in recognizing pancreatic cancer. Falling mortality rates can be due to improved treatment rather than to falling incidence rates, as is the case for large bowel cancer over the last twenty years.

All the common varieties of gastrointestinal cancers share a tendency to increase in frequency with age, tumours being rare before the age of forty but rising in incidence logarithmically thereafter.

The patterns observed are likely to be due primarily to environmental rather than to genetic factors, and this conclusion receives compelling support from comparisons of cancer incidence and mortality data obtained in migrants. Thus, the Japanese who have moved to California develop cancer incidence rates which tend to parallel those of the native born Americans, with a reduced incidence of gastric cancer and a raised frequency of large bowel cancer.

Interpretation of estimates of cancer frequency

Most varieties of alimentary cancer cause death in a high proportion of affected individuals, this being particularly true for oesophageal, gastric and pancreatic cancer. Death rates may therefore be acceptable as alternatives to incidence rates. Cancer of the large intestine by contrast causes death in some three-quarters of affected individuals and general clinical evidence suggests that the proportions of people with operable and curable disease has risen as time has passed.

Even if death rates are equivalent to incidence rates, the figures are still subject to vagaries of certification practice. Such problems are particularly likely in the elderly, and in those with cancer which may be more difficult to diagnose with certainty. Even with cancer of the stomach, accuracy of certification may be surprisingly poor, and this is illustrated by an analysis of certification accuracy carried out in London (Table 3.1).[1] The final balance in this study

Table 3.1 Extent of agreement or disagreement between clinicians' diagnoses of alimentary cancer and autopsy findings.[1]

Cancer site	Total number of clinical diagnoses	Total number of autopsy diagnoses	Total number of correct clinical diagnoses
Oesophagus	75	74	53
Stomach	253	234	148
Colon	200	175	82
Rectum	88	89	59
Pancreas	78	96	40

between the total numbers of cancers of the stomach and other disease was virtually equal, but the overall figures contain large counter weighting components of gastric cancer ascribed to other disease, and other disease ascribed to gastric cancer.

The frequency of common cancers increases steadily in a logarithmic fashion with age and therefore age-specific incidence rates, or overall incidence rates standardized for age are needed to give a true picture of the frequency of the disease.

If standardized rates are used then the age pattern of the standardizing population will affect the apparent incidence rates. African populations, for instance, contain a high proportion of younger people and therefore a standard population based upon the African distribution will underestimate for the frequency of cancer which predominantly affects the elderly.[2,3] Tables 3.2 and 3.3 show the effects of different standardizing rates upon measured standar-

Table 3.2 Standard populations used in calculating age-standardized incidence rates.[2] (Figures abridged.)

Age	Number in population (thousands)		
	African	European	World
0–19	40	29	40
20–39	40	28	28
40–59	15	27	21
60+	5	16	11

Table 3.3 Variations in age-standardized incidence rates in men per 100 000 for gastric cancer according to standardization method.[2]

	African	European	World
Japan, Miyagi	46·8	123·6	84·6
Finland	19·3	56·8	37·5
UK, Birmingham	12·0	34·8	23·3
USA, Connecticut	7·1	20·7	13·5
Rhodesia, Bulawayo	5·1	11·8	8·2

dized incidence rates for gastric cancer. The incidence rates found vary by almost three-fold when measured by different techniques, but the order for incidence rates remains unchanged from area to area. Use of different standardizing methods will affect the apparent relative frequency of cancers if they occur in age groups which achieve greater or lesser weighting by those methods. Thus, if primary liver cancer as a disease of young adults is compared with gastric cancer as a disease of the elderly, then their relative frequency will vary according to the standardizing methods.

In general, if detailed consideration is to be given to cancer frequency then age-specific incidence rates should be used rather than age-standardized rates. Standardized rates nevertheless form a convenient means of comparing cancer frequency from place to place. In this chapter, European rates have been used for standardization, since they are usually better known.

Oesophageal cancer

Epidemiologically it has been usual to separate tumours of the upper, middle and lower thirds of the gullet. Hypopharyngeal tumours tend to have different behavioural patterns from other neoplasms of the oesophagus, but there are no sound reasons for believing that cancers of the middle and lower thirds of the gullet differ materially in cause or behaviour. Most oesophageal tumours are squamous in type; adenocarcinomata which occur at the gastro-oesophageal junction are generally assumed to originate from the stomach, but occasional adenocarcinomata can be found which arise in the gullet, and which are clearly well above the gastro-oesophageal junction. They presumably originate from the mucous glands which can be detected in the oesophagus.

Incidence

There is probably a greater variation in frequency from low to high incidence areas than is found with any other tumour. Evidence about the incidence of oesophageal cancer tends to be reasonably reliable. Clinically, the progressive and remorseless dysphagia of oesophageal cancer is not paralleled by the behaviour of any other disease. Sophisticated radiological or endoscopic services therefore do no more than confirm what is clinically obvious. Furthermore, few oesophageal tumours are treated successfully, and in consequence incidence and mortality rates are almost identical. Estimates of tumour frequency therefore tend to be soundly based even in areas with rudimentary medical services, provided that patients seek help and that cancer registries collect reasonably comprehensive data.

Table 3.4 shows some of the world-wide variation in the frequency of oesophageal cancer. Oesophageal cancer is probably very common

Table 3.4 Cancer of the oesophagus. Age standardized incidence rates in men and women per 100 000 and male to female ratios in selected areas.[3]

	Men	Women	Ratio
Rhodesia, Bulawayo: African	111·3	54·0	2·1
South Africa, Cape Province: Bantu	54·2	18·2	3·0
Coloured	14·1	0·0	—
White	9·5	1·5	6·3
Japan: Miyagi Prefecture	21·7	7·5	2·9
Okayama Prefecture	6·4	3·4	1·9
USA: Hawaii: Hawaiian	21·3	0·0	—
Caucasian	8·0	1·8	4·4
Connecticut	8·2	2·0	4·1
Europe: Finland	10·2	7·8	1·3
Yugoslavia, Slovenia	9·3	1·9	4·9
Poland, Warsaw	7·7	2·8	2·8
UK, Birmingham	7·2	4·0	1·8
Norway	4·3	1·5	2·9

44 Gastrointestinal cancer

in a belt which extends from the South Caspian Sea across Asia into China and is probably very common in certain parts of tropical Africa such as Kenya as well as Rhodesia. The fifty-fold or greater variation which occurs is, however, a patchy phenomenon and in Africa, on the South Caspian littoral (Fig. 3.1) and probably

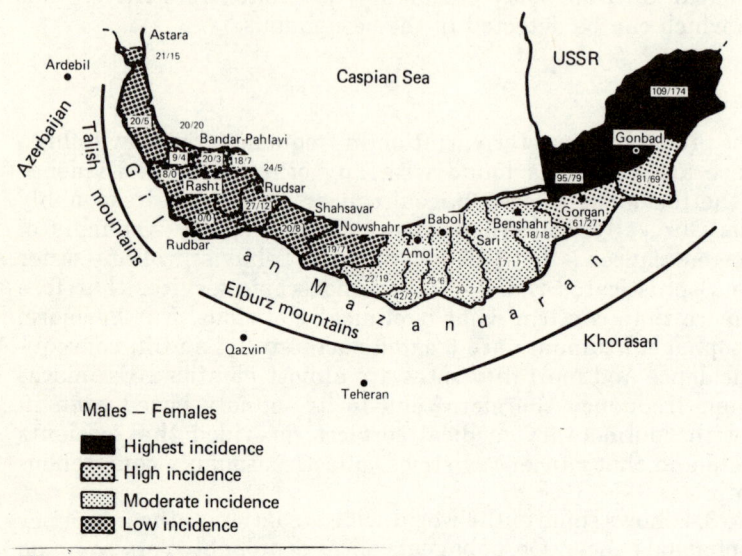

Fig. 3.1 Incidence of eosophageal cancer on the South Caspian littoral.[4] Figures denote the age standardized incidence rates for cancer of the oesophagus in men and women respectively. (Reproduced from *Science*. Copyright 1972 by the American Association for the Advancement of Science.)

elsewhere in Asia, disease frequency fluctuates greatly, a phenomenon which should make it easier to understand the underlying causal factors.[2-6] In Europe oesophageal cancer is relatively infrequent; it tends to follow the same variation as does liver cirrhosis,[7,8] presumably because of a common association with alcohol consumption. Incidence rates do not correlate with those for any other tumour, including gastric cancer, and again in contradistinction to gastric cancer there is a large variation in male to female incidence ratios, due in part to an association with alcohol consumption.

Age incidence Like other gastrointestinal cancers, oesophageal cancer tends to increase in frequency logarithmically after the age of 40, before which age it is rare (Fig. 3.2). This pattern of increase is seen universally, and there are no age groups which are otherwise peculiarly susceptible or immune Such a pattern is consistent with cancer induction after prolonged exposure to an environmental agent or agents or with a long latent period.

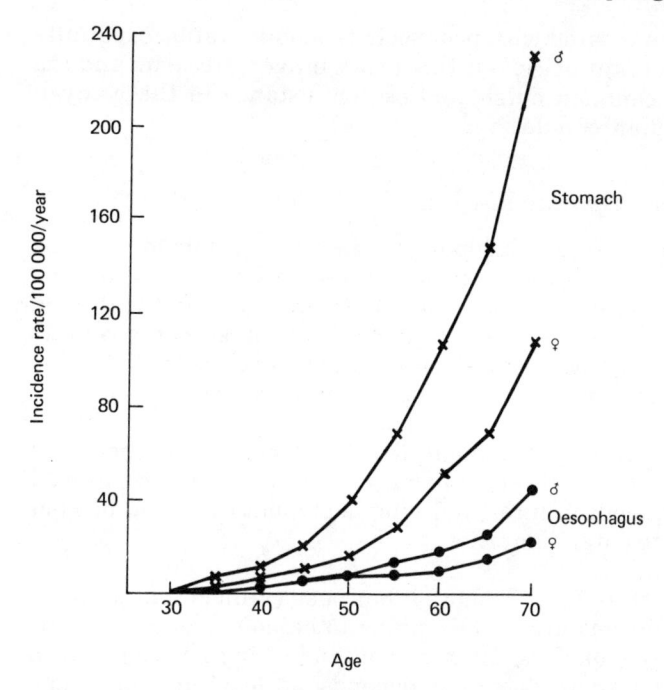

Fig. 3.2 Cancer of the stomach and eosophagus in England (Birmingham region) Age-specific incidence rates 1963–66

Sex incidence In almost all areas oesophageal cancer is commoner in men than in women, but this pattern is variable. Within Europe the male predominance is probably most marked in those places where the cancer is most common, presumably where alcohol consumption is an important factor. However, a male predominance is not necessarily observed in all high incidence areas, and the sex ratio is almost equal in the South Caspian area which has one of the highest incidence rates yet recorded.

Time trends Within Europe oesophageal cancer frequency does not seem to have changed materially with time, but the figures available only cover a short period. By contrast, oesophageal cancer has probably increased greatly in frequency in certain areas in Southern Africa. The reasons are unclear, but there does seem to be an association with a change from a rural to an urban pattern of existence, and this with living at a low economic standard.

Occupational factors No particular working group seems to be especially prone to oesophageal cancer, except those such as bartenders, who have the easiest access to alcohol. Oesophageal cancer is in some areas associated with poor socio-economic status, especially within urban communities, but this is not universally true and the disease can be common outside cities, for instance in the Kenyan and South Caspian populations.

Associated or predisposing diseases

Achalasia of the cardia   Oesophageal cancer is common and has been detected in 15% or more of patients with achalasia. The tumours are squamous in type and tend to occur within the dilated segment about the oesophageal sphincter. This presumably reflects cancer induction by the stagnant oesophageal contents. Relief of the achalasia does not prevent the development of cancer.

Coeliac disease   Initial data suggested that there was an increased frequency of oesophageal cancer in patients with this disease as well as a raised frequency of intestinal lymphoma, but the trend has not been observed in later figures.

Hiatus hernia and reflux   Though it has been claimed that patients with these conditions are unduly prone to oesophageal cancer, the evidence is not compelling. Both hernia and reflux are common in the elderly, and their detection depends at least in part upon enthusiastic perseverance by the radiologist. One reason for believing that abnormalities of the gastro-oesophageal junction do not predispose to oesophageal cancer is that such cancers are not unduly common in those with symptoms of reflux which are sufficiently severe to justify surgery.

Iron deficiency   Clinically the significance of the Patterson-Kelly (Plummer-Vinson) syndrome in predisposing to upper oesophageal cancer has long been appreciated. The mechanism is unclear.

Tylosis   In rare families this congenital disorder in which there is hyperkeratosis of the palms of the hands and of the soles of the feet is associated with the development of oesophageal cancer as a dominantly inherited disorder. Why this should happen in a few such families but not in the others is not understood.

Predisposing factors

Our knowledge of the factors associated with liability to oesophageal cancer is somewhat better than our understanding of those associated with liability to other types of cancer, but we still have little understanding of the major factors. Those who smoke and/or who drink alcohol are more liable to oesophageal cancer than those who do not, but the underlying factors which contribute to these associations are obscure. Outside these associations our knowledge is rudimentary.

Alcohol The tendency for mortality rates for hepatic cirrhosis and for oesophageal cancer to be high or low together suggests a common association. In addition retrospective case control studies have shown that European and United States patients with oesophageal cancer have stronger histories of alcohol consumption even after standardization for smoking habits (Table 3.5) than do patients with

Table 3.5 Relative risk of oesophageal cancer in relation to alcohol consumption after standardization for smoking habits.[14]

Units of alcohol	Beer	Whisky
Less than 1	0·4	0·3
1–6	1·5	1·6
6 or more	2·6	6·4

(1 unit = 1 oz of whisky or 8 oz of beer: data are for smokers of 18–34 cigarettes per day).

other varieties of cancer or control individuals without cancer.[8,14] A similar association between alcohol consumption and liability to oesophageal cancer can be found in tropical Africa,[10] but the link is not universal. Alcohol does not seem to be consumed by the population living on the South Caspian littoral where oesophageal cancer is probably at least ten times as frequent as in France. Further evidence that alcohol is unlikely to be an important factor on the south side of the Caspian Sea is that men and women tended to be affected equally often, and much of the male predominance for oesophageal cancer in other areas is probably attributable to alcohol intake.

The nature of the substance or substances associated with alcohol consumption which predispose to oesophageal cancer is not known. Alcohol itself may be an important promoting factor, but alcoholic beverages contain a large variety of ill-characterized substances which may well be of greater significance. Oesophageal cancer seems to be especially frequent in France in Brittany, and this has been ascribed to the consumption of Calvados, a liquor based upon a cider distillate. Again, in Central Africa the contamination of distilled spirits by nitrosamines has been claimed to be an important factor, though the analytical evidence upon which this assertion was based has since been contested.[9-11] By contrast, in Kenya there is epidemiological evidence to suggest that the association is strongest with maize beer drinking, whilst beer brewed from bananas, millet or sorghum is relatively trouble-free.[12]

Tobacco Cancer of the oesophagus, like cancer of the lung and of the bladder tends to be more frequent in smokers than in non-smokers. Furthermore, the risk of oesophageal cancer seems to increase with the amount smoked. Smoking and drinking tend to be associated habits and it is therefore hard to decide which of the habits is the more important.[14-16] However Table 3.6 shows that

Table 3.6 The effect of smoking on the incidence of lung and oesophageal cancer in British doctors. Annual death rate per 100 000 men, age standardized.[16]

	Non-smokers	Current smokers, any tobacco (g/day)		
		1–14	15–24	≤25
Lung	10	52	106	224
Oesophagus	3	12	13	30

there is a distinct risk gradient for oesophageal cancer in relation to smoking habits, though one which is less pronounced than for lung cancer.

Dietary factors Liability to oesophageal cancer has never been shown to be associated with any specific dietary factor. Theoretically, the large variations in oesophageal cancer frequency over short distances should make it easier to throw light upon the causal factors, but efforts have been poorly rewarded so far. The problems are illustrated by comparison of the geographical, cultural and other features of the low and high incidence districts on the South Caspian littoral. The former contain farming communities living on fertile soils which support a range of crops and a population which is, in consequence, well nourished and relatively affluent.[4] The latter tend to live in places where the soil is of poor quality, often of high salinity and therefore where the range of crops is limited and the resulting output is of poor quality. As a natural consequence all comparisons between such districts yield clear contrasts and there is no means of knowing which is of critical importance. The alternative method of comparing the cultural and other characteristics of people within high incidence areas, or within low incidence areas, who have and have not developed cancer has proved equally unhelpful. Epithelial tissues depend upon certain trace nutrients for proper growth, and lack of two in particular, vitamin A and zinc ions can be shown to be associated with dysplasia or poor renewal. However, there is no further evidence to suggest that lack of these or any other substances is an important determinant of liability to oesophageal cancer.

Nitrosamines are known to be potent carcinogens,[13] and there have been repeated suggestions that they may be important inducers of oesophageal and other cancers in man. Preformed nitrosamines have been detected in extremely low concentrations in foods such as smoked fish, but they have not been consistently and clearly detected in alcoholic drinks. Nitrosamines can also be formed in the body by the interaction of secondary amines and nitrites in the presence of acid, and the possible significance of these in relation to gastric cancer is discussed later (p. 55). So far, nitrosamine carcinogenesis remains a theoretical rather than a proven entity.

Carbohydrate food grains grown on poor soils such as those which are zinc-deficient are claimed to be prone to fungal disease, and maize has been claimed to be affected by *Aspergillus* growth in these circumstances with a resulting production of aflatoxins which are powerful carcinogens.[17,18] Again, direct proof of this theoretical pathway has yet to be obtained.

Proof of the importance of individual dietary factors by epidemiological methods seems likely to be hard to obtain. Retrospective dietary histories are unsatisfactory because patients' recall is poor and their memories are likely to be biased by the possession of alimentary disease. Prospective studies are impractical because disease incidence is low and we do not know what is the critical interval between aetiological event and tumour appearance. Broad comparisons of habits between affected and trouble-free areas have so far failed and there is no reason for believing that later attempts are likely to be more successful. It is therefore hard to see what epidemiological step it is logical to take.

Gastric cancer

Almost all tumours are adenocarcinomata, with varying degrees of differentiation from one patient to another, and also from one site to another within the tumour. Some have histological or histochemical characteristics which suggest an origin within areas of intestinal metaplasia and it has been proposed that intestinal types tend to occur in areas where gastric cancer is relatively common, possibly in association with a widespread propensity to atrophic gastritis.[19] So far, however, there has been no other reason found for believing that causal factors differ materially in patients with intestinal and non-intestinal types of tumour. Lymphomata and sarcomata occasionally develop in the stomach, but these are so few that they can safely be ignored epidemiologically.

Incidence

In general the frequency of gastric cancer varies gradually from one

50 Gastrointestinal cancer

area to another. Incidence rates tend to be high in Japan, Iceland and some parts of South America. They also tend to be relatively high in Eastern Europe, to fall progressively with change in latitude westwards, and they are very low in the USA and Canada.[2,3] Table 3.7 gives some comparative figures, and from these it can be seen

Table 3.7 Cancer of the stomach. Age-standardized incidence rates in men and women per 100 000 and male to female ratios in selected areas.[2]

	Men	Women	Ratio
Japan, Miyagi Prefecture	136·0	62·8	2·2
Colombia, Cali.	82·6	35·8	2·3
Puerto Rico	43·4	19·0	2·3
USA, Hawaii: Hawaiian	65·2	34·6	1·9
Caucasian	25·5	13·0	2·0
Connecticut	22·6	10·7	2·1
Canada, Newfoundland	56·6	34·0	1·7
Quebec	23·1	10·2	2·3
Yugoslavia, Slovenia	67·7	35·8	1·9
Finland	67·3	36·2	1·9
Poland, Warsaw	54·0	25·6	2·1
Germany, Hamburg	57·6	27·0	2·1
Norway	44·1	24·0	1·8
Denmark	42·7	26·3	1·6
UK, Birmingham	37·6	20·2	1·9

that the frequency varies ten- to twenty-fold between high and low risk areas. Incidence rates can vary significantly within countries, thus there are regional variations described within Czechoslovakia, and rates in North Wales are double those within the rest of the United Kingdom.

In places where incidence data are not available, mortality rates can be substituted since they are almost equivalent in most parts of the world, provided that death certification and coding practices are accurate. The assumption that this is always true in highly developed countries is not necessarily reasonable, since gastric cancer has sometimes in the past been used more as an acceptable legal criterion for interment than as an accurate medical opinion about the cause of death. The growing emphasis upon the early detection of gastric cancer as a means of lowering mortality does not so far seem to have affected the virtual equivalence of mortality and incidence data, probably because the proportion of small tumours detected remains very small.

Age and sex incidence Gastric cancer frequency increases progressively with advancing age in men and women (Fig. 3.2). No differences in overall pattern are detectable between countries with high and low incidence rates. All increase steadily with age but the figures for low incidence areas are consistently lower than those found in high incidence areas.

Approximately twice as many men as women develop gastric cancer. This imbalance is constant, and the sex ratio does not change materially with advancing age, nor between high and low incidence areas. The proportion of men and women does, however, seem to differ according to tumour site. Cancer of the gastric antrum appears to be equally common in women and men, but cancer of the fundus to be about twice as common in men as in women. The change in sex ratio according to tumour site suggests that causal influences differ.[20] One obvious possibility would seem to be that fundal neoplasms tend to occur in smokers, but the excess mortality of smokers with cancer seems to be fully accounted for by cancer of the respiratory tract, the mouth, pharynx, oesophagus and bladder. A further possibility is that any excess of men with fundal cancer is simply due to misclassification of lower oesophageal squamous cancer as gastric adenocarcinoma.

Time trends Gastric cancer incidence rates have tended to change variably in different parts of the world. Thus, whilst figures were falling in the USA there was, until recently, a tendency towards an increase in Japan, though this has probably been reversed now. Indirect measurement of incidence rates by examining mortality rates in the United Kingdom suggest that incidence rates, which were static, are now falling.[21] This trend is brought out by a comparison of mortality experience in men born in successive time periods [cohort mortality] (Fig. 3.3).[21] The underlying reasons are not understood. They may at least in part be due to an association with poverty in an urbanized population.

Occupational and social factors There is a pronounced socio-economic gradient in liability to gastric cancer. This is well illustrated by comparative data on mortality according to social class collected by the Registrar General in England and Wales. Gastric cancer now seems to be at least three times as common in unskilled people as in the professional and managerial groups, whereas there was only about a two-fold difference in the past (Table 3.8).[22] The cause of these changes is not understood. Examination of incidence rates within individual working groups does not suggest any outstanding differences between them, except for a possible association with work in mining, in rubber industries, and with asbestos.[100]

52 Gastrointestinal cancer

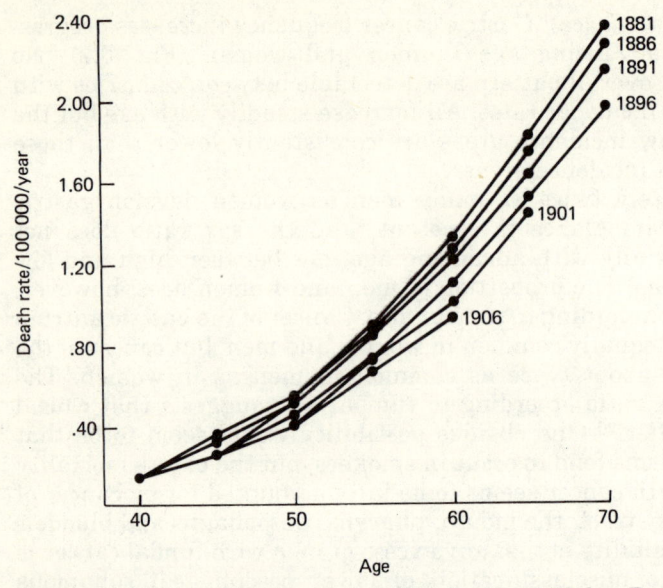

Fig. 3.3 Cancer of the stomach in England and Wales. Death rate by **age** according to year of birth 1881–1906[21]

Table 3.8 Standardized mortality ratios for cancer of the stomach in England and Wales.[22]

Year	Social class				
	I	II	III	IV	V
1921–23	60	82	100	106	130
1930–32	55	83	98	112	122
1950	57	67	100	114	132
1961	49	63	101	114	163

Associated diseases

Pernicious anaemia Patients with pernicious anaemia have a three- to four-fold increase in their chances of developing gastric cancer. This change is independent of the association between blood group A and liability to pernicious anaemia or to gastric cancer.[23]

Atrophic gastritis The development of chronic atrophic gastritis but not superficial gastritis alone is associated with an increased liability to gastric cancer. The risk is probably equivalent to that of patients with pernicious anaemia. As in pernicious anaemia it seems likely that the gastric atrophy increases general susceptibility to prevailing environmental influences.

Gastric resection Though some have suggested that patients who have had resections for benign ulceration are at increased risk of developing cancer, others have denied this. In a matched control study five times the expected frequency was detected, and clinical results tend to confirm that the risk is increased. Gastric juice nitrite levels have been found to be raised after gastrectomy suggesting that nitrosamine formation may be important.[94-96]

Gastric ulcer Gastric ulceration is often observed at the edge of carcinomata and in consequence it has been suggested that ulceration predisposed to cancer formation. Follow-up studies of ulcer patients in fact show that the risk of cancer does not differ materially from that of normal people of the same age and sex. Any apparent increase in the risk of malignancy supervening in ulcer patients is probably attributable to initial misdiagnosis.[25]

Genetic predisposition

Gastric cancer is more common than would have been expected by chance in the families of gastric cancer or pernicious anaemia patients, a difference which is small but distinct. At least part of the increase could be due to improved recall of the disease in family members and to the operation of common environmental factors, but this cannot be the whole explanation. Gastric cancer is about 20% commoner in people of blood group A than in those of the remaining blood groups, a difference which is yet unexplained. Mucous secretions are rich sources of blood group substances but a variable effect of these upon cancer liability seems unlikely. Blood group substances are present superficially in mucosal cells or in secretions according to the individual's blood group and also according to whether the individual can secrete these substances in water soluble form or not, a separately inherited genetic characteristic. Even in individuals who are non-secretors a variable blood group effect is detectable.

Environmental predisposing factors

Comparisons of gastric cancer frequency in migrants with their expected disease incidence if they had stayed in their native country show that rates tend to change to match those of their adopted land.[26] Thus, Japanese who settle in California have gastric cancer incidence rates which are part way between those of their native and adopted lands, but they fall to the level of their new country in the second generation. This change could be due in whole or part to a slow alteration of life patterns or to a long time span over which environmental influences work.

At present we do not know what factors influence gastric cancer incidence. The biggest demonstrable difference in the United Kingdom, and probably in most other Western countries, lies in the differential incidence between the affluent and the poor, but poverty itself is an imprecise label.

Diet No specific dietary item has been associated with later liability to gastric cancer. This lack of evidence springs from the difficulties inherent in conducting satisfactory case control comparisons, with the problems of dietary recall and in deciding what interval may be necessary for factors to act as particular important difficulties. Table 3.9 illustrates the unreliability of answers about culinary and dietary habits in periods three decades earlier.[27]

Table 3.9 Reproducibility of pairs of answers by stomach cancer and control patients to questions about dietary habits 25 years earlier.[27]

	Complete agreement	Partial or complete disagreement	Incomplete or inapplicable answers
Spread used most often on bread	36·5	46·0	17·5
Fat used most often in cooking	41·6	37·5	20·8
Metal from which saucepans were made	43·7	43·7	12·5
Metal from which frying pans were made	33·3	52·0	14·6

Correlation analysis has been substituted for such studies, with broad comparisons of dietary intake and average cancer incidence within different countries being used to identify possible important factors. Such figures have been used to suggest that gastric cancer is common where protein intake is low, or almost equivalently where carbohydrate foods are the most important sources of energy. Further suggestions have been made of specific links with potato consumption and with low vitamin intake such as of vitamin C in fresh vegetables. Such analyses have proved difficult to refine further, and themselves have defects in their methods.[28] The importance of the correlations detected depends greatly upon the extent to which corrections are made for the variable contributions of other factors. Thus an initial positive correlation for one factor can appear unimportant or even to be reversed if one or two other dietary items are included in a correlation matrix.

Alcohol Gastric cancer incidence does not seem to be affected by consumption of alcohol either as simple beers and wines or as fortified spirits.

Smoking Tobacco consumption does not seem to be a significant cause of gastric cancer.

Dietary contaminants and specific dietary items The consumption of smoked foods has frequently been suggested as a cause of gastric cancer in Iceland, and carcinogens such as benzpyrene have been suggested as the important factors. However, benzpyrene does not appear to cause adenocarcinoma, though it will induce squamous cancer. Substances which will induce adenocarcinomata include aflatoxins[29] and nitrosamines.[13] The former have been discussed already as potential causes of oesophageal cancer: theoretically they could also cause gastric cancer but no satisfactory evidence of a link has yet been obtained.

Nitrosamines are powerful carcinogens and could be ingested preformed, and trace amounts below those required for carcinogenesis in experimental animals, but not necessarily for long-term effects in man, have been detected in some foods.[30] An alternative source lies in the interaction of nitrites and secondary amines in the stomach. Nitrites are commonly used in food preservation, and secondary amines can be found where food is imperfectly preserved. Thiocyanates, which are present in gastric juice and saliva, will catalyse this reaction, as will bacteria.[24,34,40–42] Evidence available to support a nitrosamine carcinogenesis hypothesis is circumstantial. Patients with pernicious anaemia have very high gastric juice nitrite concentrations and simulation studies *in vitro* suggest the volatile nitrosamines could be generated.[92] At least two studies have suggested that gastric cancer is unduly common in areas where the water supply contains large amounts of nitrate (from which nitrite could be formed).[31,35] Furthermore, vitamin C will inhibit the reaction of nitrosation[32] and a negative correlation has been found between liability to gastric cancer and green vegetable consumption.[33] By contrast, the role of thiocyanates as important promoters of nitrosamine formation and hence cancer induction in the stomach must be doubtful, for if they possessed such properties then one might expect smokers, who have high plasma and salivary thiocyanate levels, to be especially prone to gastric cancer. More evidence is required before the role of nitrosamines as inducers of gastric cancer is accepted, in the same way that their significance as cancer inducers elsewhere needs stronger support.

Trace metal imbalance has been suggested as a possible important factor in the increased frequency of gastric cancer in North Wales.[36] A relative disproportion of zinc to copper ratios has been found in the soil[37] but why this should influence cancer incidence (if it does), is obscure. An alternative explanation which has been propounded has been that brackens which grow on relatively acid soils, as in North Wales, contain carcinogenic principles which could enter the water supply. Again, this proposition suffers from lack of direct support.[38,39]

Small intestinal cancer

Less than a hundredth of the total incidence of gastrointestinal cancer is due to neoplasms of the small bowel. Apart from knowledge about some of the diseases which predispose to small bowel cancer our understanding of its causes is virtually nonexistent.

Adenocarcinoma

There is an increased risk of small intestinal adenocarcinoma in Crohn's disease. However, this risk, though detectable, is very small, and is less than a tenth of the risk of large bowel cancer in patients with ulcerative colitis.

Carcinoid tumours

These can arise anywhere in the gut, and also outside it, for instance in the ovary and lung. The classical metastasizing tumour which causes diarrhoea and flushing is usually due to a tumour with primary origin in the small gut. The reason why such tumours occur is not understood, as with all the other rare varieties of endocrine tumours of the gut.

Lymphoma

Lymphoid tumours of the small bowel are a recognized complication of coeliac disease.[43,44] The increase may be related to the lymphoid and plasma cell infiltrate which is always demonstrable in the submucosa. One hypothesis explaining the basis of coeliac disease postulates that there is a hypersensitivity to gluten. The constant immune stimulation associated with such a phenomenon could then lead to spontaneous over-activity and multiplication within the lymphoid series. Patients with familial Mediterranean fever also have an increased risk of lymphoid over-reactivity, the causes being unclear.

The reasons why the small intestine is rarely a site of cancer incidence are unknown. Crypt cells are buried deep in the mucosa and are therefore relatively protected from the external environment. However, exactly the same could be said of the pancreas where cancer is much more common.

Large intestinal cancer

This is one of the commonest varieties of cancer in Western communities; histologically virtually all cancers of the large intestine are adenocarcinomata. Cancer tends to occur more frequently in the caecum, sigmoid colon and rectum than elsewhere, and a distinct division is usually accepted between colonic and rectal cancer. For epidemiological purposes it is doubtful whether there is, in fact, any fundamental distinction between the two sites. The situation is further complicated by the fact that the division takes place within a region of relatively high cancer frequency which lacks a clear demarcation line between the sigmoid colon and rectum. In practice it is therefore difficult to decide whether a difference in frequency of sigmoid and rectal cancer between two population groups reflects a real difference or is simply due to variations in classification. Further separation can also be made between cancer of the caecum and ascending colon, the transverse colon and flexures and the descending colon. Again, this separation has as yet made little contribution to our understanding of the causes of large bowel cancer.

Incidence

Tables 3.10 and 3.11 compare some of the recorded incidence rates in Europe and elsewhere. In general the figures for cancer of the

Table 3.10 Cancer of the colon. Age-standardized incidence rates in men and women per 100 000 for areas listed in Table 3.7 for gastric cancer.[2]

	Men	Women	Ratio
Japan, Miyagi Prefecture	5·8	5·8	1·0
Colombia, Cali.	4·9	6·2	0·8
Puerto Rico	7·2	8·9	0·8
USA, Hawaii: Hawaiian	31·8	19·5	1·6
Caucasian	28·6	40·8	0·7
Connecticut	41·0	40·5	1·0
Canada, Newfoundland	29·1	26·8	1·1
Quebec	23·1	23·6	1·0
Yugoslavia, Slovenia	8·2	7·6	1·1
Finland	9·9	10·9	0·9
Poland, Warsaw	8·9	10·1	0·9
Germany, Hamburg	19·1	19·5	1·0
Norway	18·2	17·6	1·0
Denmark	24·1	26·6	0·9
UK, Birmingham	23·0	22·1	1·0

58 Gastrointestinal cancer

Table 3.11 Cancer of the rectum. Age-standardized incidence rates in men and women per 100 000 for areas listed in Table 3.7 for gastric cancer.[2]

	Men	Women	Ratio
Japan, Miyagi Prefecture	6·9	7·3	1·0
Colombia, Cali.	5·4	4·0	1·4
Puerto Rico	5·4	5·8	0·9
USA, Hawaii: Hawaiian	8·6	10·0	0·9
Caucasian	18·2	14·3	1·3
Connecticut	24·2	15·8	1·5
Canada, Newfoundland	16·6	10·9	1·5
Quebec	15·8	10·7	1·5
Yugoslavia, Slovenia	12·1	8·8	1·4
Finland	11·6	9·6	1·2
Poland, Warsaw	8·1	5·6	1·4
Germany, Hamburg	16·8	12·7	1·3
Norway	10·3	7·0	1·5
Denmark	26·1	15·7	1·7
UK, Birmingham	23·9	13·8	1·7

colon and rectum tend to run in parallel except for the tendency for rectal cancer to be more frequent in men and colonic cancer to be commoner in women. The incidence of large bowel cancer is high in Western communities and low outside them, and in general within Western countries there tends to be an inverse correlation between the frequency of large bowel and stomach cancer. Thus, there is a high incidence of large bowel cancer in North America, where stomach cancer is relatively uncommon, and frequencies are lower in Japan and Finland, where stomach cancer is more common. Migrants from Japan to the USA adopt the cancer incidence patterns of their host country within one generation, suggesting a potent environmental influence whose nature remains obscure.[26]

Age and sex incidence Both cancer of the colon and cancer of the rectum become more common with advancing age, like other gastrointestinal cancers (Fig. 3.4). Although rectal cancer is more frequently a disease of men and colonic cancer a disease of women, there is, in fact, a change in the sex ratio with advancing age. Roughly equivalent proportions of men and women develop rectal cancer at the ages of 40 to 50 years, but by the age of 60 there are about twice as many men as women with rectal cancer.[47,48] By contrast, there is a markedly greater proportion of women than men with colonic cancer at the age of 40, but by the age of 60 this difference has virtually disappeared (Fig. 3.5). The change in sex ratio with advancing age which is observed with these two types of cancer is not found with any other variety of gut cancer.

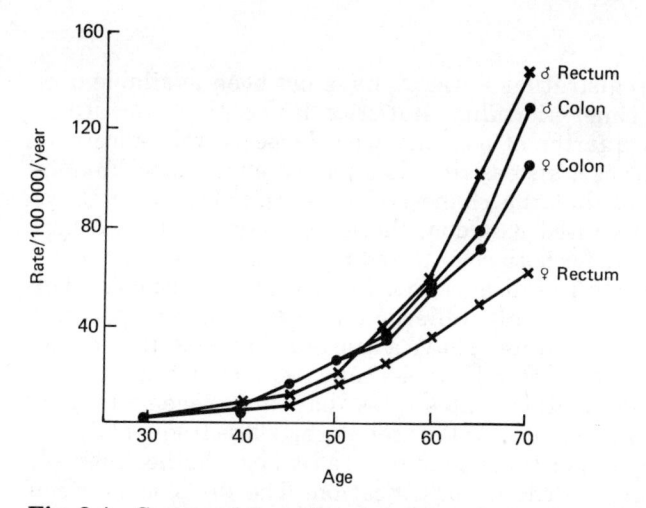

Fig. 3.4 Cancer of the colon and rectum in England (Birmingham region) Age-specific incidence rates 1963–66[2]

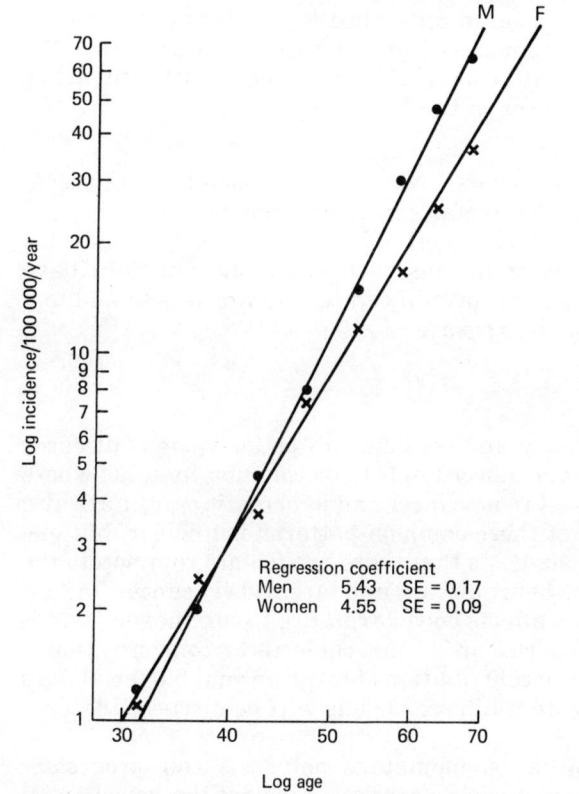

Fig. 3.5 Cancer of the rectum in England and Wales 1961–62

Gastrointestinal cancer

Time Trends

Reliable cancer registration statistics have not been available over long periods of time. Mortality statistics make poor substitutes because up to a quarter of patients with large bowel cancer are cured of their disease; also as time has passed surgical techniques have improved, so that the chances of successful treatment have improved. In the United Kingdom there has been a fall in cohort mortality with time for both colonic and rectal cancer (Figs. 3.6 and 3.7),[21] but this trend has disappeared for more recent cohorts. The earlier fall almost certainly reflects improvements in operative techniques which are failing to have a continued impact. In addition the frequency of large bowel cancer may be increasing in some areas. Thus, in the United States intestinal cancer seems to have become more common and rectal cancer slightly less frequent.[91] It is hard to be sure whether these changes are real or whether they are due to a progressive drift in classification. The division between colonic and rectal cancer is made at a high incidence area, the sigmoid colon, so that a small change in the line at which a division was made could make a large difference to the apparent relative frequency of the two tumours. Clinical experience confirms the suggestion that there may be a real change in the relative frequency of colonic and rectal cancer in the USA.[97]

Occupational and social factors   No particular social class is especially prone to colonic or rectal cancer. In the past it has been suggested that the relatively well off are more likely to develop colonic cancer, but any trend has been small. Recent data have suggested an increased susceptibility in textile workers to add to a possible association with exposure to asbestos.[98,99]

Associated diseases

Comparisons of mortality and incidence rates for various diseases suggest that large bowel cancer tends to be common in areas where coronary heart disease, breast cancer and pancreatic cancer are also common.[45] The basis of these common patterns is unclear, but one prevalent hypothesis suggests that there are factors common to the production of coronary heart disease and large bowel cancer, in that dietary fibre deficiency affects bowel exposure to carcinogens and is also associated with a rise in serum cholesterol concentration.[46] This hypothesis, and the contribution of intraluminal bacterial flora to the production of potential carcinogens will be discussed later.

Colonic polyps   Familial adenomatous polyposis coli progresses inevitably to overt metastasizing carcinomatosis if the bowel is not resected prophylactically. The significance of solitary benign polyps is less clear, but the following general propositions seem to be true. The general distribution of solitary adenomatous polyps within the bowel seems to parallel that of cancer (Table 3.12).[46,49] The age

Table 3.12 Localization of benign polyps and of large intestinal carcinomata in Malmö, Sweden.[49]

Site	Percentage distribution	
	Polyps	Cancers
Caecum and ascending colon	23·2	17·6
Transverse colon and flexures	14·6	11·4
Descending colon	10·0	4·3
Sigmoid colon	25·2	31·0
Rectum	19·9	35·6
Uncertain	7·0	0·1
Total number	954	1198

distribution of patients with polyps is similar to that of patients with large bowel cancer, and polyps tend to be rare in countries where large bowel cancer is also rare. The true risk of cancer developing within polyps is unknown, since most are resected when found because of the risk that they may become malignant. Whatever the strength of direct association, it seems that the factors which predispose to solitary adenomatous polyp formation and to overt cancer are similar if not identical.

Ulcerative colitis and Crohn's disease Patients with non-specific ulcerative colitis who have extensive disease involving the bowel from the rectum and proximally beyond the splenic flexure are at increased risk of developing cancer of the colon. This risk only becomes apparent once the disease has been present for at least ten years, the chances of malignant change being variously estimated at one in ten and one in four if the colon is left *in situ* indefinitely. A curious feature of the cancer which complicates colitis is its tendency to develop more commonly in the proximal colon than would be expected if malignancy were occurring in an ordinary non-colonic population, and this despite the fact that colitis always involves the rectum, and the rest of the colon to a variable extent.[47]

There is also probably an increased risk of colonic cancer in patients with Crohn's disease, but this is probably much less than that in ulcerative colitis. Exact figures determining the risk in Crohn's colitis are impossible to obtain because the distinction between classical ulcerative colitis and Crohn's colitis is not absolute, the one grading clinically and histologically into the other.

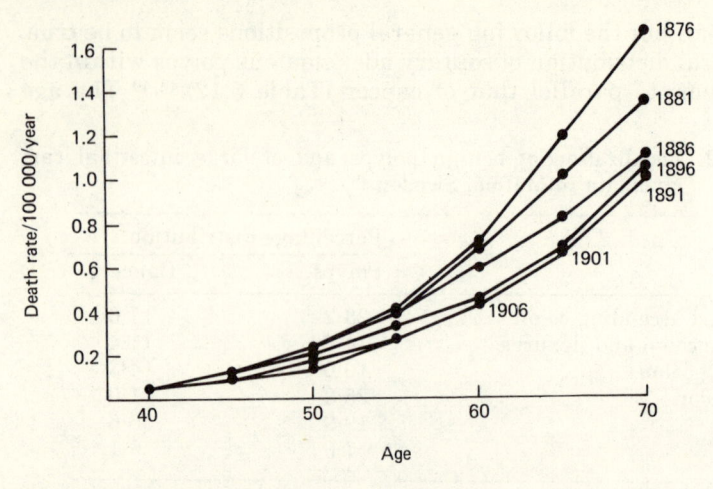

Fig. 3.6 Cancer of the intestines in England and Wales. Death rate by age according to year of birth 1876–1906[21]

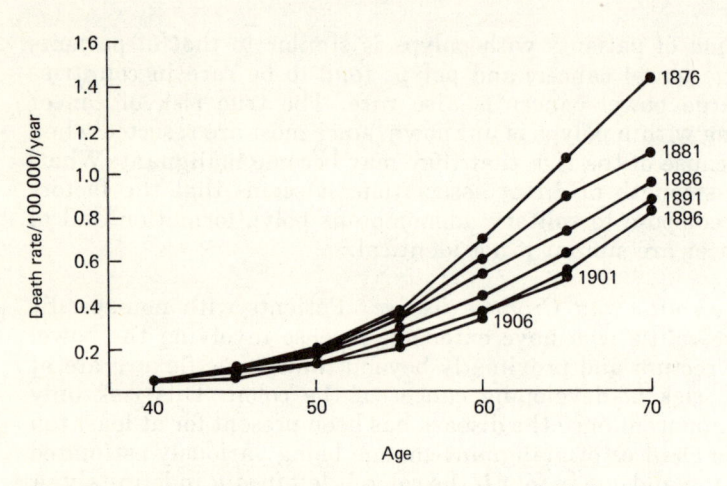

Fig. 3.7 Cancer of the rectum in England and Wales. Death rate by age according to year of birth 1876–1906[21]

Environmental predisposing factors

Smoking has generally been found to have no influence upon liability to colonic and rectal cancer, but correlations between consumption patterns and cancer mortality rates in the USA, together with secular and other trends, suggest an association between beer drinking and liability to large intestinal and particularly rectal cancer.[50] Any mechanism for the association which is supported by some, but not by others, is unclear.

Greater attention has been paid to general dietary characteristics, particularly intakes of beef and fat. Though correlations between beef and fat intake and liability to colo-rectal cancer have been repeatedly suggested from national consumption correlation patterns and dietary analyses, the general epidemiological evidence is equivocal. Thus analyses of beef and fat consumption patterns in the USA and India have failed to support the beef or fat associations suggested, and some case control studies in the USA and Scandinavia have likewise shown no association between consumption of these dietary items and the occurrence of colo-rectal cancer.[51-57]

Despite the inconsistencies of the evidence, there are some supporting data from metabolic and animal studies suggesting that diets, particularly those rich in beef, can modify bacterial flora in the gut and bile acid excretion patterns in ways which could increase liability to large bowel cancer.[59] Bile acids bear structural similarities to carcinogenic polycyclic hydrocarbons, and in experimental animals lithocholic and taurodeoxycholic acids act as tumour promoters for cancer induction by 1,2-dimethylhydrazine.[58]

Comparisons of the faecal flora of normal populations living in high and low colonic cancer incidence areas have also given some support to this hypothesis. The proportions of anaerobic bacteria such as *Bacteroides* species in the faeces of populations living in the United Kingdom and the United States have been found to be relatively high, whilst aerobic species were more prevalent in faecal samples obtained in Uganda, Japan and India. Anaerobic bacteria are also in general more capable of metabolizing bile acids than are aerobic bacteria, and a particularly close correlation has been found between faecal concentrations of dihydroxycholanic acids, probably mostly derived from deoxycholate, and the incidence of colonic cancer.[59,60,62]

Table 3.13 shows one set of data comparing faecal bacterial output

Table 3.13 Effect of diet upon faecal characteristics.[61,62]

	Mixed Western diet	Non-meat diet
Total anaerobes (Log_{10}/g dry wt)	11·5 ± 0·1	11·1 ± 0·1
β-glucuronidase (μg phenolphthalein hydrolysed per hour)	35 ± 3·8	10 ± 1·4
Total neutral sterols (mg/g dry wt)	28·2 ± 1·7	19·1 ± 3·6
Total bile acids (mg/g dry wt)	12·9 ± 0·8	11·1 ± 0·9

and activity and bile acid concentrations in healthy people taking normal mixed and meat-free diets.[61] Though total anaerobic bacterial concentrations did not change, their activity altered as measured by glucuronidase activity and the proportion of neutral sterols increased together with glucuronidase activity on the mixed diet. By contrast when another population of healthy people were given high or low fat diets, faecal bacterial flora and glucuronidase activity were unaltered though faecal bile acid concentrations rose when animal fat intake was raised.[93]

The pathways by which bacterial activity could promote cancer induction are unclear, but Fig. 3.8 illustrates some theoretical

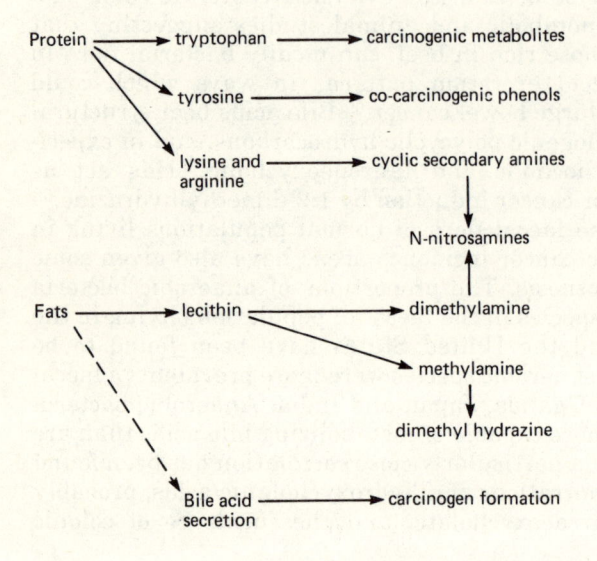

```
Protein ──────► tryptophan ──────────► carcinogenic metabolites
        ╲
         ╲──► tyrosine ──────────────► co-carcinogenic phenols
          ╲
           ╲► lysine and ────────────► cyclic secondary amines
              arginine                         │
                                               ▼
                                         N-nitrosamines
                                               ▲
Fats ──────► lecithin ───────────────► dimethylamine
     ╲                    ╲
      ╲                    ►methylamine
       ╲                         │
        ╲                        ▼
         ╲                dimethyl hydrazine
          ╲
           ►Bile acid ──────────► carcinogen formation
            secretion
```

Fig. 3.8 Theoretical possible mechanisms of carcinogenesis in the colon[63]

mechanisms.[63] Direct supporting evidence is lacking but, for instance, a high glucuronidase activity could result in deconjugation of bile acids which might be an important initial step before their conversion to other active metabolites.

There is also a body of contrary evidence, thus, when a group of prospective coronary heart disease studies were analysed it was found that, if anything, those with lower serum cholesterol concentrations developed colon cancer more frequently.[64] In addition a high protein intake in volunteers was found to have little if any effect upon faecal bacterial flora in at least one study.[65] Finally, a comparison of dietary intakes and faecal characteristics in a high colonic cancer incidence area in Scandinavia from Denmark and a low incidence area from Finland failed to confirm a relationship between nuclear dehydrogenating clostridia found previously, nor one with faecal steroid output, though differences were observed in the faecal populations of non-sporing anaerobes, bacteroides and eubacteria.[53]

Parallel with and interdigitating with this bile acid hypothesis is another which proposes that dietary fibre deficiency is of basic importance. It is suggested that the incidence of large bowel cancer is inversely related to the consumption of unabsorbable fibre. Fibre could contribute to protecting against bowel cancer in several ways. Firstly, the bulky stools produced by those who consume unabsorbable fibre would tend to dilute any carcinogens, and secondly, the bowel transit time would be reduced, thus reducing the contact period available in the large bowel. Thirdly, dietary fibre itself could beneficially alter the intraluminal bacterial flora, though it should be remembered that the dietary fibre is heterogeneous and the type and source can alter its effect.[66]

Further support for the bile acid/fibre hypothesis comes from studies showing that, when analysed retrospectively, the proportion of dietary fibre is reduced in those who develop colonic cancer compared with control individuals.[67]

Some of these data have been contested, thus the Japanese who live in Hawaii, and who have bowel cancer incidence rates similar to those of the indigenous American population, have appreciably faster gut transit times, whilst the Japanese in Japan have identical transit times with the Japanese living in Hawaii, but a lower colon cancer risk (Table. 3.14).[68]

Table 3.14 Bowel transit, stool weight and frequency of bowel movements in residents of Hawaii and Japan.[68]

	USA (Hawaii) Caucasian	USA (Hawaii) Japanese	Japan (Akita) Japanese
Mean bowel transit time (hours)	56·2	31·4	33·9
Mean stool weight (grams)	119·7	120·7	194·7
Mean interval between bowel actions (hours)	21·7	20·1	22·8
Colonic cancer risk	High	High	Low

So far no bile acid product has been shown to cause adenocarcinoma rather than other varieties of cancer; however, it is becoming increasingly clear that the heterogeneous group of substances which comprise dietary fibre are neither functionally nor metabolically inert. Further evidence is needed to confirm their role in protection against cancer induction.

Other factors Obesity, constipation and the use of laxatives have all been associated with liability to colonic cancer,[69] but the strength and importance of these is unclear, partly because analyses have rested upon retrospective studies of earlier life patterns and the reliability of responses must be doubtful, and partly because mechanisms may not be directly through the agents studied.

Pancreatic cancer

Adenocarcinomata of the pancreas are common tumours, and they arise predominantly from ductular tissue. Endocrine tumours and the rare ampullary tumours are so comparatively few that broad epidemiological examination of the features of all pancreatic cancer taken as a whole is essentially the epidemiology of ductular disease.

Incidence

The frequency of pancreatic cancer tends to be greater in European countries and in North America than elsewhere, but the correspondence with incidence patterns of, for instance, colonic cancer, is indifferent (Tables 3.10 and 3.15), as with those for degenerative arterial disease. Areas with low frequencies so far recorded include parts of Africa, India and Singapore. Since very few tumours are

Table 3.15 Cancer of the pancreas. Age-standardized incidence rates in men and women per 100 000 for areas listed in Table 3.7 for gastric cancer.[2] Other areas with recorded incidences below 3·0 per 100 000 India (Bombay), Nigeria (Ibadan), Singapore (Malays and Indians).

	Men	Women	Ratio
Japan, Miyagi Prefecture	9·5	5·6	1·7
Colombia, Cali.	3·9	4·6	0·8
Puerto Rico	7·8	4·9	1·6
USA, Hawaii: Hawaiian	20·9	20·1	1·0
Caucasian	10·6	7·9	1·4
Connecticut	12·1	6·7	1·8
Canada; Newfoundland	9·2	4·3	2·1
Quebec	7·3	4·4	1·7
Yugoslavia, Slovenia	5·7	3·8	1·5
Finland	11·8	7·9	1·5
Poland, Warsaw	11·0	7·4	1·5
Germany, Hamburg	11·3	6·5	1·7
Norway	11·0	5·8	1·9
Denmark	10·3	7·1	1·5
UK, Birmingham	10·8	5·9	1·8

resectable, mortality tends to be equivalent to incidence. However, accurate statistics still depend upon high post mortem examination rates since the diagnosis when simply based on clinical patterns or even investigations is frequently wrong. Despite these problems it seems likely that the disease is indeed rare in countries which are in general underdeveloped, although the relatively high frequency in developed areas may correspond at least in part with medical sophistication.

Pancreatic cancer increases steadily in frequency with age, like other gastrointestinal tumours, and it is also slightly more common in men than in women. No particular patterns of variation with age or sex are discernible in any special areas.

Time trends Since the diagnosis of pancreatic cancer depends upon sophisticated techniques or upon high autopsy rates, it is difficult to know whether any apparent increase in prevalence of pancreatic cancer is attributable to a true rise in incidence or to improving medical diagnostic services. However, the recorded frequency of pancreatic cancer has doubled or trebled in the United Kingdom and the USA over the last thirty years, whilst a quadrupling of frequency has been noted in Japan. The extent to which such changes reflect diagnostic transfer from, for instance, cancer of the stomach, with increasing precision or sophistication of diagnosis, is totally unclear. The increasing cohort mortality shown in Fig. 3.9 for England and Wales could reflect either a true incidence change, since most patients die, or else a rise in the use of the clinical diagnosis which had previously been under-used.

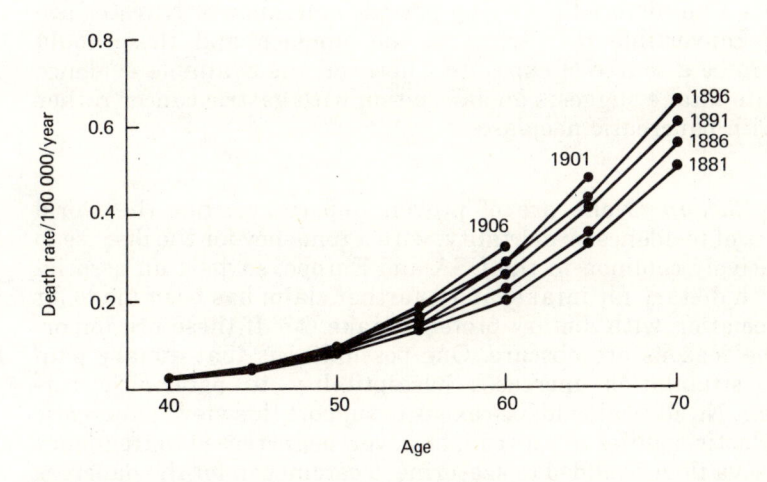

Fig. 3.9 Cancer of the pancreas in England and Wales. Death rate by age according to year of birth 1881–1906[21]

Associated diseases

Diabetes mellitus has consistently been found to be associated with an increased liability to pancreatic cancer, the neoplasm making itself evident many years after diagnosis of the diabetes.[76] The increase in frequency is approximately a doubling and its reasons are uncertain. No association with chronic pancreatitis has ever been detected.

Environmental predisposing factors

Occupational and social No clear patterns of occupational and social factors have emerged: an association with work in the chemical industry has been detected, though this could represent diagnostic activity in workers receiving good medical care. Any tendency for the disease to be more common in the relatively well-off could similarly be accounted for by diagnostic bias as well as by any real difference in incidence, and such problems bedevil the interpretation of all statistics.

The pancreas is protected by the duodenal mucosa from direct contact with the luminal environment of the gut and therefore any carcinogen presumably acts after absorption. So far we have no knowledge as to what factors may be important.[71]

Certain carcinogens, notably the nitrosamines, are known to be capable of inducing cancer at sites remote from those where they have been administered. Methylnitrosourea is one such substance. Proof of exposure to such substances in amounts which will cause cancer is probably impossible to obtain, since the influence of trace amounts administered over long periods is unknown. Nitrates are readily convertible to nitrites in the stomach and these could therefore be a source of exposure. However, the available evidence of nitrate intake suggests an association with gastric cancer rather than with pancreatic neoplasms.

Dietary factors None are of proven importance, but the world patterns of incidence or mortality, with a tendency for the disease to be relatively common in the USA and Europe, suggest an association with dietary fat intake, and a further claim has been made for an association with dietary protein intake.[70,72] If these are important the reasons are obscure. One possibility is that dietary pancreatic stimulation increases susceptibility to pancreatic carcinogens. No clinical evidence exists to support this view: pancreatic hyperplastic nodules in rats can, however, be increased in frequency if raw soya flour is added to azaserine, a carcinogen for the pancreas in rats, perhaps due to pancreatic hyperplastic responses to the trypsin inhibitory component present in the soya flour.[73]

Smoking A series of studies have suggested an association between liability to pancreatic cancer and smoking,[74,75] but interpretation is difficult. A direct causal relationship may not hold because a dose response with number of cigarettes smoked has not always been detectable. In addition, the tendency to smoke may be associated with other possibly important factors such as alcohol consumption, though this has never been proven to induce pancreatic cancer rather than pancreatitis.

Hepatic cancer

Primary tumours of the liver can appear to be predominantly cholangiolar or hepatocellular in origin. International classifications do now provide for distinction between these two patterns.

Incidence

Primary liver cancer is rare in developed countries, but high incidences are found in underdeveloped areas (Table 3.16), particu-

Table 3.16 Cancer of the liver. Age-standardized incidence rates in men and women per 100 000 in selected areas.[2]

	Men	Women	Ratio
Japan, Miyagi Prefecture	1·7	1·1	1·5
Colombia, Cali.	6·0	6·2	1·0
Puerto Rico	3·6	2·2	1·6
USA, Hawaii: Hawaiian	21·2	5·5	3·8
Caucasian	6·6	2·9	2·3
California: white	3·7	1·5	2·5
negro	12·9	1·9	6·8
Canada, Saskatchewan	1·6	1·4	1·1
Yugoslavia, Slovenia	2·5	1·5	1·7
Finland	1·8	1·1	1·6
Poland, Warsaw	4·7	1·1	4·2
Norway	2·4	0·6	4·0
Denmark	3·4	2·7	1·3
UK, Birmingham	1·0	0·4	2·5
Bulawayo: African	90·0	36·0	2·5
Cape Province: Bantu	35·1	10·8	3·3
coloured	2·1	0·9	2·3
white	1·6	0·8	2·0
Nigeria, Ibadan	13·4	5·2	2·6

larly in Southern Africa where liver and oesophageal cancer seem to be the predominant varieties. Primary liver cancer is common in parts of Rhodesia, South Africa, Kenya and Uganda, where it is basically a disease of the native African population.[77,78]

Gastrointestinal cancer

Within Africa itself the frequency of liver cancer varies markedly, thus incidence rates are reported to be particularly high in Lourenço Marques, and distinctly lower in Johannesburg and Kampala (Table 3.17). In European communities liver cancer mainly arises in

Table 3.17 Primary liver cancer: proportionate rates of hepatoma in Africa.[78]

	Liver tumours as percentage of all tumours
Rhodesia	11·3
Lambarene (Gabon)	9·7
Shirati (Tanzania)	7·9
Uganda	6·8
Kenya	5·2
Tanzania	3·0
Sudan	1·6

association with hepatic cirrhosis. Men are at greater risk of this tumour than women; in Western communities this may simply be a measure of their greater tendency to abuse alcohol. In Africa the male predominance is probably less marked. No specific age group seems to be at special risk of liver cancer, the frequency probably increasing steadily with advancing age. Clear time trends in incidence have not been recognized. In Western countries this may simply be because of the overall rarity of primary liver cancer, whilst in Africa it could be because cancer registries have only developed relatively recently. Differences in apparent frequency of liver cancer in Western countries have to be examined with caution, secondary hepatic involvement is many times more common than primary disease and misallocation clinically or in coding between primary and secondary disease could greatly affect figures.

Occupational factors One rare variety of tumour, hepatic angiosarcoma, is an occupational risk in those who manufacture vinyl chloride.[79,80]

Associated diseases

Hepatic cirrhosis Primary liver cell cancer (as opposed to cholangiocarcinoma) complicates cirrhosis in 10 to 15% of patients. The cause of the cirrhosis seems to be irrelevant, and cancer has been recorded as complicating haemochromatosis, idiopathic cirrhosis and alcoholic liver disease. The relative risk of cancer in cirrhotics in different countries is difficult to calculate; some evidence suggests that hepatic or post-necrotic cirrhosis may confer a great risk of liver cancer than alcoholic cirrhosis, but confident comparisons are hard to make in the absence of clearly defined at-risk populations.

Hepatitis B virus infection Patients with hepatocellular carcinoma have frequently been found to have hepatitis B surface or core antigen in their serum,[90] and there is a strong suggestion that virus infection predisposes to hepatoma, presumably by inducing chronic active hepatitis and then cirrhosis. However it is equally likely that co-carcinogenic factors (such as aflatoxins) are necessary for hepatoma to occur, and it is possible, though unlikely, that the development of hepatocellular carcinoma activates latent hepatitis B virus.

In Africa it has been suggested that nutritional liver disease predisposes to the development of liver tumours, but this lacks confirmation. Hepatic abnormalities in kwashiorkor are rapidly correctable, and no visible hepatic changes then remain. Difficulties arise in assessment because kwashiorkor, infectious hepatitis and cirrhosis, and liver cancer may be common in the same areas.[81] This does not necessarily mean that they are all related causally. In particular, cirrhosis may well be a rare event to complicate long-standing kwashiorkor, and simple protein deficiency probably plays, at best, a minor role in the development of cirrhosis. There is experimental evidence to suggest that the protein-deficient liver is particularly susceptible in experimental animals to the general toxic properties of aflatoxin, but this may not hold for the carcinogenic properties.

Drugs

Despite the fact that the liver is an important route for drug detoxication, virtually no drugs in ordinary use have been shown to cause liver cancer in man. The risk of primary hepatic tumours does, however, seem to be increased in those who take very large doses of anabolic steroids,[84] it is also possible, and indeed likely, that drugs such as oxyphenisatin which can cause chronic active hepatitis may through this indirectly lead to liver cancer if cirrhosis becomes established. *N*-acetyl-2-aminofluorine, and amino-azo compounds such as dimethylaminoazobenzene are carcinogenic; and nitrosamines and aflatoxins may be important carcinogens in man.[85,86] These last two groups of compounds are discussed elsewhere (p. 49).

Oral contraceptives have been associated with the development of hepatic tumours: lesions usually consist of adenomata or areas of focal nodular hyperplasia but malignant tumours have been encountered. If there is a true association it is likely to be very infrequent, thus no such tumours were detected during over 51 000 patient-years of treatment in one study in the United Kingdom.[82,83]

Environmental predisposing factors

Parasitic infestations There seems good reason for believing that infection with *Clonorchis sinensis* will predispose to the development of cholangiolar cancer, and the same may be true for *Schistosoma mansoni*. Such disease will not however account for the pattern of liver cancer throughout the tropics, including high frequencies in the Chinese, firstly because the frequency of the parasitic diseases does not mirror liver cancer incidence, and secondly because hepatocellular cancer does not occur as a direct consequence of parasitic disease, only bile duct cancer.

Plant toxins The best example of a plant used as a foodstuff which is hepatotoxic is the cycad nut. Cycasin (methylazo-oxymethanol-β-D-glucoside) as the aglycone is clearly carcinogenic in animals. The nut meal contains cycasin as a non-toxic glycoside, but hydrolysis, which could be carried out by gut bacterial flora, to the aglycone, could lead to the formation of a highly active methylating agent, similar to that in dimethylnitrosamine. However, there is no reason for believing that this or any other naturally derived plant product is the main cause of tropical liver cancer, though certain naturally occurring substances such as the pyrrolizidine alkaloids, derived from *Senecio* species amongst others, are carcinogenic in animals.

Fungal toxins Clear proof that fungal contamination is an important cause of tropical liver cancer has yet to be obtained but there are strong indicators that it may be important.

In Africa there is an association between poverty and the development of liver cancer. Poorer people there tend to depend heavily upon cereal based foods, and these are liable to fungal contamination. *Aspergillus* species, particularly *Aspergillus flavus*, grow on cereals harvested and stored under poor conditions, and aflatoxin is a potent hepatic carcinogen. Furthermore, aflatoxin has been isolated from foods sampled in Uganda where hepatoma is a comparatively common disease.

Cancer of the gallbladder and bile ducts

Cancer of the gallbladder and bile ducts is an infrequent variety of tumour. Thus in England and Wales in 1969, 550 cases of gallbladder cancer were diagnosed, together with 327 cases of extra-hepatic bile duct cancer, and 114 tumours of the ampulla of Vater, 74 other tumours not having their site specified. By contrast there were 4249 diagnoses of cancer of the pancreas.[87]

Gallbladder and bile duct cancer tends to be slightly more common in women than in men, and to increase in frequency with advancing age. Age-standardized incidence rates in Western Europe and the United States range between 2·0 and 5·0 per 100 000 population per year. Outside these areas variable frequencies are recorded, but no consistent patterns are detectable. In particular, those areas with high incidences of primary liver cancer do not necessarily have high frequencies of gallbladder and bile duct cancer. In those that do, the common trend may reflect a lack of diagnostic precision in identifying primary hepatocellular and bile duct cancers rather than on true tendency towards association.

Associated diseases

Little is known of the aetiology of gallbladder or bile duct tumours, but two diseases are associated with them, gallstones (commonly) and ulcerative colitis (rarely).[88,89]

Gallstones The assumption that gallstones have a causal relationship to the development of cancer is based on the following proposition. Firstly, gallstones are found in most patients with gallbladder cancer; secondly, there is a similar male to female ratio in gallstone disease and in gallbladder cancer. Thirdly there is a tendency for both gallstones and gallbladder cancer to be common in the same geographical areas or else, as in Israel, in the same ethnic groups (Table 3.18).

Table 3.18 Gallstones and gallbladder and biliary tract cancer in Israel.[88]

	Percentage of patients with gallstones	
	Men	Women
Gallbladder cancer	69·0	89·8
Biliary tract cancer	20·0	62·5

The relationship of biliary tract cancer to the presence of gallstones is less certain, because the frequency of gallstones in patients with biliary tract cancer tends to be lower. Table 3.18 illustrates these points, showing that in patients in Israel, gallstones were present in most patients with gallbladder cancer, but in less of those with biliary tract cancer. In addition, though women born in Europe had a higher frequency of gallstones than African or Asian born women, stones were present in the same proportion with gallbladder cancer.[88]

The explanation of the association between gallstones and gallbladder cancer is unclear. No evidence is available to show that any special variety of stone is associated, nor that there is more or less likely to be evidence of chronic cholecystitis.

Inflammatory bowel disease There have been repeated case reports suggesting that patients with ulcerative colitis are prone to bile duct tumours. In one such report, eight of 103 patients with carcinoma of the proximal bile ducts proved to have had ulcerative colitis.[89] Colitis has usually been of longstanding, or else colectomy has already been performed, gallstones are seldom detected in association, and few patients seem to have had ascending cholangitis. Patients with ulcerative colitis are also prone to primary sclerosing cholangitis and it is possible that there is a common aetiology for carcinoma and for sclerosing cholangitis.

References

1. Heasman, M. A., Lipworth, L. (1966). *Accuracy of Certification of Cause of Death.* Studies on medical and population subjects. No. 20. London, HMSO.
2. Doll, R., Muir, C., Waterhouse, J. (1970). *Cancer Incidence in Five Continents Vol II.* Berlin, Springer.
3. Doll, R., Payne, P., Waterhouse, J. (1966). *Cancer Incidence in Five Continents Vol I.* Berlin, Springer.
4. Kmet, J., Mahboubi, E. (1972). Esophageal cancer in the Caspian littoral of Iran: initial studies. *Science* **175,** 846–53.
5. Co-ordinating group for research on the etiology of esophageal cancer of North China (1974). Epidemiology and etiology of esophageal cancer in North China. *Chinese Medical Journal* **11,** 189.
6. Ahmed, N., Cook, P. (1969). The incidence of cancer of the oesophagus in West Kenya. *British Journal of Cancer* **23,** 302–12.
7. Tuyns, A. (1970). Cancer of the oesophagus: further evidence on the relation to drinking habits in France. *International Journal of Cancer* **5,** 152–6.
8. Schwartz, D., Lellouch, D., Flamand, R., Denoix, P. F. (1962). Alcool et cancer. Resultats d'une enquête rétrospective. *Revue Française d'études clinique et biologique* **7,** 590–604.
9. McGlashan, N. D., Patterson, R. L. S., Williams, A. A. (1970). *N*-nitrosamines and grain-based spirits. *Lancet* **2,** 1138.
10. Collis, C. H., Cook, P. J., Foreman, J. K., Palframan, J. F. (1972). Cancer of the oesophagus and alcoholic drinks in East Africa. *Lancet* **1,** 441.
11. Gough, T. A. (1977). A search for volatile nitrosamines in East African spirit. *Gut* **18,** 301–2.
12. Cook, P. (1971). Cancer of the oesophagus in Africa. *British Journal of Cancer* **25,** 853–80.
13. Lijinsky, W., Epstein, S. S. (1970). Nitrosamines as environmental carcinogens. *Nature* **225,** 21–3.
14. Wynder, E. L., Bross, I. J. (1961). A study of etiological factors in cancer of the esophagus. *Cancer* **14,** 389–413.

15. Hammond, E. C. (1964). Smoking in relation to mortality and morbidity: findings in first thirty-four months of follow-up in a prospective study, started in 1959. *Journal of the National Cancer Institute* **32**, 1161–88.
16. Doll, R., Peto, R. (1976). Mortality in relation to smoking: 20 years' observations on male British doctors. *British Medical Journal* **2**, 1525–36.
17. Hesseltine, C. W., Shotwell, O. L., Ellis, J. J., Stubblefield, R. D. (1966). Aflatoxin formation by *Aspergillus flavus*. *Bacteriological Reviews* **30**, 795–805.
18. Burrell, R. J. W., Roach, W. A., Shadwell, A. (1966). Esophageal cancer in the Bantu of the Transkei associated with mineral deficiency in garden plants. *Journal of the National Cancer Institute* **36**, 201–9.
19. Munoz, N., Correa, P., Cuello, C., Duque, E. (1968). Histologic types of gastric carcinoma in high and low-risk areas. *International Journal of Cancer* **3**, 809–18.
20. Flamant, R., Lassevre, O., Lazar, P., Leguerinais, J., Denoix, P., Schwartz, D. (1964). Differences in sex ratio according to cancer site and possible relationship with use of tobacco and alcohol. *Journal of National Cancer Institute* **32**, 1309–16.
21. Case, R. A. M., Coghill, C., Davies, J. M., Harley, J. L., Hytten, C. A., Pearson, J. T., Willard, S. R., Alderson, M. R. (1976). *Serial Mortality Tables: Neoplastic Diseases Volume I*. Division of Epidemiology. Institute of Cancer Research, London.
22. *Registrar General's Decennial Supplements. England and Wales. Occupational Mortality 1921, 1931, 1951, 1961*. (1927, 1931, 1958, 1971). London, HMSO.
23. Blackburn, E. K., Callender, S. T., Dacie, J. V., Doll, R., Girdwood, R. H., Mollin, D. L., Saracci, R., Stafford, J. L., Thompson, R. B., Varadi, S., Wetherley Mein, G. (1968). Possible association between pernicious anaemia and leukaemia: a prospective study of 1625 patients with a note on the very high incidence of stomach cancer. *International Journal of Cancer* **3**, 163–70.
24. Ruddell, W. S. J., Bone, E. S., Hill, M. J., Blendis, L. M., Walters, C. L. (1976). Gastric juice nitrate. A risk factor for cancer in the hypochlorhydric stomach. *Lancet* **2**, 1037–9.
25. Ihre, B. J. E., Barr, H., Havermark, G. (1964). Ulcer-cancer of the stomach. *Gastroenterologia* **102**, 78–91.
26. Buell, D., Dunn, J. E. Jr. (1965). Cancer mortality among Japanese Issei and Nisei of California. *Cancer* **18**, 656–64.
27. Acheson, E. S., Doll. R. (1964). Dietary factors in carcinoma of the stomach: a study of 100 cases and 200 controls. *Gut* **5**, 126–31.
28. Armstrong, B. K., Mann, J. I., Adelstein, A. M., Eskin, F. (1975). Commodity consumption and ischaemic heart disease mortality, with special reference to dietary practices. *Journal of Chronic Diseases* **28**, 455–69.
29. Butler, W. H., Barnes, J. M. (1966). Carcinoma of the glandular stomach in rats given diets containing aflatoxin. *Nature* **209**, 90.
30. Crosby, N. T., Foreman, J. K., Palframan, J. F., Sawyer, R. (1972). Estimation of steam-volatile *N*-nitrosamines in foods at the 1 µg/kg level. *Nature* **238**, 342–3.
31. Hill, M. J., Hawksworth, G., Tattersall, G. (1973). Bacteria, nitro-

samines and cancer of the stomach. *British Journal of Cancer* **28**, 562–7.
32. Raineri, R., Weisberger, J. H. (1975). Reduction of gastric carcinogens with ascorbic acid. *Annals of the New York Academy of Sciences* **258**, 181–9.
33. Haenszel, W., Kurihara, M., Segi, M., Lee, R. K. C. (1972). Stomach cancer among Japanese in Hawaii. *Journal of the National Cancer Institute* **49**, 969–88.
34. Hawksworth, G., Hill, M. J. (1971). Bacteria and the N-nitrosation of secondary amines. *British Journal of Cancer* **25**, 520–6.
35. Correa, P., Haenszel, W., Cuello, C., Tannenbaum, S., Archer, M. (1975). A model for gastric cancer epidemiology. *Lancet* **2**, 58–60.
36. Stocks, P. (1950). Cancer of the stomach in the large towns of England and Wales. *British Journal of Cancer* **4**, 147–57.
37. Stocks, P., Davies, R. I. (1960). Epidemiological evidence from chemical and spectrographic analyses that soil is concerned in the causation of cancer. *British Journal of Cancer* **14**, 8–22.
38. Hirono, I., Shibuya, C., Fushimi, K., Haga, M. (1970). Studies on carcinogenic properties of bracken, *Pteridium aquilinum*. *Journal of the National Cancer Institute* **45**, 179–84.
39. Pamukcu, A. M., Price, J. M., Bryan, G. T. (1970). Assay of fractions of Bracken fern (*Pteris aquilina*) for carcinogenic activity. *Cancer Research* **30**, 902–5.
40. Mirvish, S. S. (1975). Formation of N-nitroso compounds: chemistry kinetics and *in vivo* occurrence. *Toxicology and Applied Pharmacology* **31**, 325–51.
41. Marquardt, H., Rufino, F., Weisburger, J. H. (1977). Mutagenic activity of nitrite-treated foods: human stomach cancer may be related to dietary factors. *Science* **196**, 1000–1.
42. Ruddell, W. S. J., Blendis, L. M., Walters, C. L. (1977). Nitrite and thiocyanate in the fasting and secreting stomach and in saliva. *Gut* **18**, 73–7.
43. Gough, K. R., Read, A. E., Naish, J. M. (1962). Intestinal reticulosis as a complication of idiopathic steatorrhea. *Gut* **3**, 232–9.
44. Holmes, G. K. T., Stokes, P. L., Sorahan, T. M., Prior, P., Waterhouse, J. A. H., Cooke, W. T. (1976). Coeliac disease, gluten-free diet, and malignancy. *Gut* **17**, 612–19.
45. Wynder, E. L., Shigematsu, T. (1967). Environmental factors of cancer of the colon and rectum. *Cancer* **20**, 1520–61.
46. Burkitt, D. (1975). Benign and malignant tumours of large bowel. *In Refined Carbohydrate Foods and Disease*, Ed. Burkitt, D. P. and Trowell, H. C. London, Academic Press.
47. Langman, M. J. S. (1967). Current trends in the epidemiology of cancer of the colon and rectum. *Proceedings of the Royal Society of Medicine* **60**, 210–12.
48. de Jong, U. W., Day, N. E., Muir, C. S., Barclay, T. H. C., Bras, G., Foster, F. H., Jussawalla, D. J., Kurihara, M., Linden, G., Martinez, I., Payne, P. M., Pedersen, E., Ringertz, N., Shanmugaratnam, T. (1972). The distribution of cancer within the large bowel. *International Journal of Cancer* **10**, 463–77.
49. Berge, T., Ekelund, G., Mellner, C., Pihl, B., Wenckert, A. (1973). Carcinoma of the colon and rectum in a defined population. *Acta chirurgica Scandinavica* suppl. 438.

50. Enstrom, J. E. (1977). Colorectal cancer and beer drinking. *British Journal of Cancer* **35**, 674–83.
51. Enstrom, J. E. (1975). Colorectal cancer and consumption of beef and fat. *British Journal of Cancer* **32**, 432–9.
52. Haenszel, W., Berg, J. W., Segi, M., Kurihara, M., Locke, F. B. (1973). Large-bowel cancer in Hawaiian Japanese. *Journal of the National Cancer Institute* **51**, 1765–79.
53. International Agency for Research on Cancer. Intestinal microecology group (1977). Dietary fibre, transit time, faecal bacteria, steroids and colon cancer in two Scandinavian populations. *Lancet* **2**, 207–11.
54. Wynder, E. L., Kajitani, T., Ishikawa, S., Dodo, H., Takano, A. (1969). Environmental factors of cancer of the colon and rectum. II. Japanese epidemiological data. *Cancer* **23**, 1210–20.
55. Higginson, J. (1966). Etiological factors in gastrointestinal cancer in man. *Journal of the National Cancer Institute* **37**, 527–45.
56. Bjelke, E. (1974). Epidemiological studies of cancer of the stomach, colon and rectum; with special emphasis on the role of diet. *Scandinavian Journal of Gastroenterology* **9**, suppl. 31, 1.
57. Bjelke, E. (1971). Case-control study of cancer of the stomach, colon and rectum. In *Oncology 1970: Proceedings of the Tenth International Cancer Congress. Vol. 5*, Ed. R. L. Clark, R. C. Cumley, J. E. McCoy, M. M. Copeland. Chicago, Year Book Medical Co.
58. Reddy, B. S., Narisawa, T., Maronpot, R., Weisburger, J. H., Wynder, E. L. (1975). Animal models for the study of dietary factors and cancer of the large bowel. *Cancer Research* **35**, 3421–6.
59. Hill, M. J., Drasar, B. S., Aries, V. C., Crowther, J. S., Hawksworth, G. M. Williams, R. E. O. (1971). Bacteria and aetiology of cancer of the large bowel. *Lancet* **1**, 95–100.
60. Hill, M. J., Drasar, B. S., Williams, R. E. O., Meade, T. W., Cox, A., Simpson, J. E. P., Morson, B. C. (1975). Faecal bile-acids and clostridia in patients with cancer of the large bowel. *Lancet* **1**, 535–8.
61. Wynder, E. L., Reddy, B. S. (1974). Metabolic epidemiology of colorectal cancer. *Cancer* **84**, 801–6.
62. Reddy, B. S., Weisburger, J. H., Wynder, E. L. (1975). Effects of high risk and low risk diets for colon carcinogenesis on faecal microflora and steroids in man. *Journal of Nutrition* **105**, 878–84.
63. Hill, M. J. (1974). Bacteria and the etiology of colonic cancer. *Cancer* **34**, 815–18.
64. Rose, G., Blackburn, H., Keys, A., Taylor, H. L., Kannel, W. B., Paul, O., Reid, D. D., Stamler, J. (1974). Colon cancer and blood cholesterol. *Lancet* **1**, 181–3.
65. Hentges, D. J., Maier, B. R., Burton, G. C., Flynn, M. A., Tsutakawa, R. K. (1977). Effect of a high-beef diet on the fecal bacterial flora of humans. *Cancer Research* **37**, 568–71.
66. Walters, R. L., McLean Baird, I., Davies, P. S., Hill, M. J., Drasar, B. S., Southgate, D. A. T., Green, J., Morgan, B. (1975). Effects of two types of dietary fibre on faecal steroid and lipid excretion. *British Medical Journal* **2**. 536–8.
67. Modan, B., Barell, V., Lubin, F., Modan, M., Greenberg, R. A., Graham, S. (1975). Low-fiber intake as an etiologic factor in cancer of the colon. *Journal of the National Cancer Institute* **55**, 15–18.

68. Glober, G. A., Nomura, A., Kamiyama, S., Shimada, A., Abba, B. C. (1977). Bowel transit-time and stool weight in populations with different colon-cancer risks. *Lancet* **2**, 110–11.
69. Boyd, J. T., Doll, R. (1954). Gastrointestinal cancer and the use of liquid paraffin. *British Journal of Cancer* **8**, 231–7.
70. Lea, A. J. (1967). Neoplasms and environmental factors. *Annals of the Royal College of Surgeons of England* **41**, 432–7.
71. Wynder, E. L. (1975). An epidemiological evaluation of the causes of cancer of the pancreas. *Cancer Research* **35**, 2228–33.
72. Ishii, K., Nakamura, K., Takeuchi, T., Hirayama, T. (1973). Chronic calcifying pancreatitis and pancreatic carcinoma in Japan. *Digestion* **9**, 429–37.
73. Morgan, R. G. H., Levison, D. A., Hopwood, D., Saunders, J. H. B., Wormsley, K. G. (1977). Potentiation of the action of azaserine on the rat pancreas by raw soya bean flour. *Cancer Letters* **3**, 87–90.
74. Hirayama, T. (1967). *Smoking in Relation to the Death Rates of 295 118 Men and Women in Japan*, p. 14. Tokyo, National Cancer Center, Research Institute.
75. Best, E. W. R. (1960). *A Canadian Study of Smoking and Health*, pp. 65–86. Ottawa, Department of National Health and Welfare.
76. Kessler, I. I. (1970). Cancer mortality among diabetics. *Journal of the National Cancer Institute* **44**, 673–86.
77. Alpert, M. E., Hutt, M. S. R., Davidson, C. S. (1968). Hepatoma in Uganda. A study in geographic pathology. *Lancet* **1**, 1265–7.
78. Hutt, M. S. R. (1971). Epidemiology of human primary liver cancer. In *Liver Cancer. Proceedings of a working conference*. I.A.R.C., Lyon.
79. Lee, F. I., Harry, D. S. (1974). Angiosarcoma of the liver in a vinyl-chloride worker. *Lancet* **1**, 1316–18.
80. Thomas, L. B., Popper, H., Berk, P. D., Selikoff, I., Falk, H. (1975). Vinyl-chloride-induced liver disease. From idiopathic portal hypertension (Banti's syndrome) to angiosarcomas. *New England Journal of Medicine* **292**, 17–22.
81. Anthony, P. P., Vogel, C. L., Sadikali, F., Barker, L. F., Peterson, M. R. (1972). Hepatitis associated antigen and antibody in Uganda: correlation of serological testing with histopathology. *British Medical Journal* **1**, 403–6.
82. Klatskin, G. (1977). Hepatic tumours: possible relationship to use of oral contraceptives. *Gastroenterology* **73**, 386–94.
83. Kay, C. R. (1976). Liver-cell adenomas and oral contraceptives. *Lancet* **2**, 52–3.
84. Johnson, F. L., Feagler, J. R., Lerner, K. G., Majerus, P. W., Siegel, M., Hartmann, J. R., Thomas, E. D. (1972). Association of adrogenic-anabolic steroid therapy with development of hepatocellular carcinoma. *Lancet* **2**, 1273–6.
85. Wogan, G. N. (1973). Aflatoxin carcinogenesis. In *Advances in Cancer Research VII*, p. 309. New York, Academic Press.
86. Alpert, M. E., Davidson, C. S. (1969). Mycotoxins. A possible cause of primary cancer of the liver. *American Journal of Medicine* **46**, 325–9.
87. Registrar General's Statistical Review of England and Wales for the three years 1968–70. Supplement on Cancer (1975). London, HMSO.
88. Hart, J., Modan, B., Shani, M. (1971). Cholelithiasis in the aetiology of gall bladder neoplasms. *Lancet* **1**, 1151–53.

89. Ross, A. P., Braasch, J. W. (1973). Ulcerative colitis and carcinoma of the proximal bile ducts. *Gut* **14**, 94–7.
90. Editorial (1978). Link between hepatoma and hepatitis. *British Medical Journal* **2**, 718–19.
91. Devesa, S. S., Silverman, D. T. (1978). Cancer incidence and mortality trends in the United States, 1935–74. *Journal of the National Cancer Institute* **60**, 545–71.
92. Ruddell, W. S. J., Bone, E. S., Hill, M. J., Walters, C. L. (1978). Pathogenesis of gastric cancer in pernicious anaemia. *Lancet* **1**, 521–3.
93. Cummings, J. H., Wiggins, H. S., Jenkins, D. J. A., Houston, H., Jivraj, T., Drasar, B. S., Hill, M. J. (1978). Influence of diets high and low in animal fat on bowel habit, gastrointestinal transit time, fecal microflora, bile acid, and fat excretion. *Journal of Clinical Investigation* **61**, 953–63.
94. Stalsberg, H., Taksdal, S. (1971). Stomach cancer following gastric surgery for benign conditions. *Lancet* **11**, 1175–7.
95. Schrumpf, E., Serck-Hanssen, A., Stadaas, J., Aune, S., Myren, J., Osnes, M. (1977). Mucosal changes in the gastric stump 20–25 years after partial gastrectomy. *Lancet* **11**, 467–9.
96. Schlag, P., Wonka, W., Meyer, H., Feyeraband, G., Merkle, P. (1977). Bakterielle besiedlung und nitritbildung im magen nach gastroenterostomie. *Langenbecks Archiv für Chirurgie* **344**, 109–14.
97. Snyder, D. N., Heston, J. F., Meigs, J. W., Flannery, J. T. (1977). Changes in site distribution of colorectal cancer in Connecticut, 1940–1973. *Digestive Diseases* **22**, 791–7.
98. Vobecky, J., Devroede, G., Lacaille, J., Watier, A. (1978). An occupational group with a high risk of large bowel cancer. *Gastroenterology* **75**, 221–3.
99. McDonald, J. C., McDonald, A. D., Gibbs, G. W. (1971). Mortality in Chrysotile asbestos mines and mills of Quebec. *Archives of Environmental Health* **22**, 677–86.
100. Haas, J., Schottenfeld, D., Lipkin, M., Good, R. A. (Eds). (1978). *Epidemiology of Gastric Cancer in Gastrointestinal Tract Cancer*. New York, Plenum.

4
Chronic non-specific inflammatory bowel disease

Chronic inflammatory disease of the small and large intestine varies in type and frequency from place to place and probably from time to time. The most important and frequent varieties are, in Western countries of unknown cause, ulcerative colitis and Crohn's disease. By contrast, tuberculous and amoebic disease are commonly observed in tropical and sub-tropical countries where non-specific varieties are infrequently described. Other varieties, including ischaemic disease and distinct sub-categories such as eosinophic enteritis and Whipple's disease are relatively rare in all countries.

Crohn's disease

The description by Crohn and his colleagues of chronic inflammatory, non-tuberculous disease predominantly of the terminal ileum dates back less than 50 years, but there seems little doubt that the disease did occur earlier although it was not distinguished from ordinary tuberculous enteritis. Later, largely following the descriptions of Morson and his colleagues[1] it was realized that Crohn's disease could simultaneously or exclusively affect the large bowel and occasionally developed higher in the gut.

This developing awareness of the range of clinical pattern of Crohn's disease has made it extremely difficult to decide if an apparently increasing incidence rate reflected a true rise in frequency, or was simply due to improvements in diagnostic standards.

Incidence and time trends

Irrespective of changes in patterns of clinical practice and diagnosis there has been general agreement that the disease is being increasingly frequently seen at least in Northern European countries. Thus data from Scandinavia, Switzerland, England and Scotland show a common rising trend either in total diagnoses or else in hospital admission rates. The same pattern has not been described elsewhere, but the discrepancy probably has three causes. In some countries systems of health care do not provide statistics about the frequency of diseases other than cancer. In other countries, such as

India or those of tropical Africa, the disease may be so rare that no interest is likely to be taken in it. Thirdly, there may be countries where Crohn's disease is prevalent but where the frequency is not rising or is only doing so slowly.

Table 4.1 Average annual incidence and prevalence rates for Crohn's disease per 100 000 population

		Incidence	Prevalence
England, Oxford[2]	1951–60	0·8	9·0
USA, Baltimore[3]	1960–63	1·8	
Scotland, Aberdeen[4]	1955–68	2·0	32·5
England, Nottingham[5]	1958–72	2·0	26·5
Norway, general survey[6]	1964–69	1·1	
Switzerland, Basle[7]	1960–69	1·6	
Denmark, Copenhagen[8]	1960–70	1·3	
Sweden, Malmö[9]	1958–73	4·3	57·0
Sweden, Uppsala and Vastmanland[10]	1968–73	5·0	50·0

Table 4.1 compares the incidence and prevalence rates of Crohn's disease recorded in nine surveys in Europe and North America. The figures are broadly comparable except that incidence rates recorded in earlier years tend to be lower than those found in later periods. Data from outside Northern Europe are fragmentary. Clinical impressions are that Crohn's disease is rare or non-existent in much of India, Africa and South America, but difficulties of interpretation arise because in any area where infective disease including tuberculosis and amoebiasis is common, and where in addition medical services are ill-developed, the chances of recognizing non-specific inflammatory bowel disease must be low.

In the USA several large groups of patients have been collected but since the populations from whom they have been drawn are undefined, there is no means of converting the figures to incidence rates. The Baltimore, Maryland, study suggests that Crohn's disease is likely to be as common as in Northern Europe but there is a lack of supporting data. In Australia Crohn's disease is well recognized but no epidemiological data are available. The same is true for Southern Europe, where the paucity of clinical reports suggests that the disease is in fact rare.

In Nottingham a detailed survey[5] showed that Crohn's disease was being diagnosed at least five times as often as ten years before, and similar rises have been recorded in Scotland, in England generally and in Scandinavia. Figure 4.1 contrasts the rising rates in England, as admissions adjusted for the effect of re-admissions so as to make them similar to incidence rates, with the incidence rates

82 *Chronic non-specific inflammatory bowel disease*

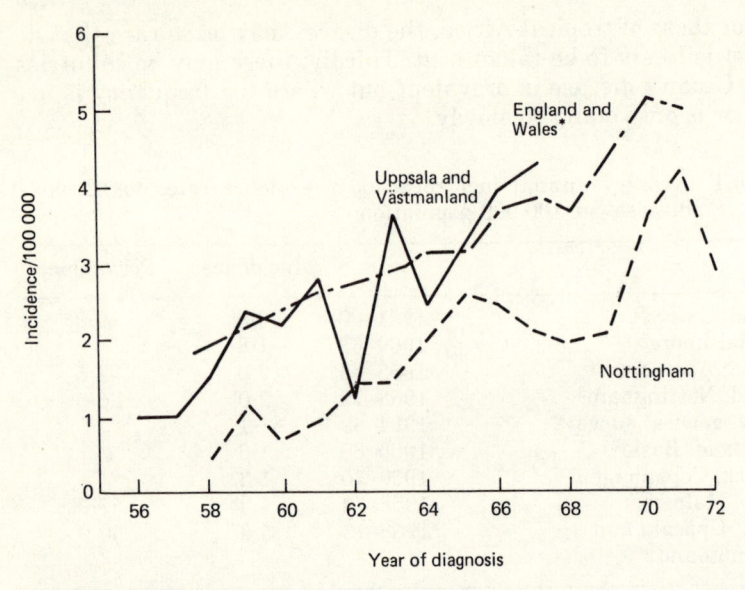

Fig. 4.1 The incidence of Crohn's disease in England and in Sweden[10] recorded in Nottingham[5] and in Uppsäla and Vastmanland,[10] Sweden. The trends are broadly comparable.

An increasing frequency of admission for Crohn's disease could plausibly be ascribed to diagnostic transfer from the category of ulcerative colitis. Little evidence exists to confirm or deny this suggestion, and what exists is contradictory, thus Kyle,[4] having found an increasing frequency of Crohn's disease in north-eastern Scotland, noted that the rise was predominantly due to the finding of more such disease in the large bowel, and concluded that diagnostic transfer could well be important. An increase in diagnoses of colonic disease was also found by Bergman and Krause in Sweden.[10] We likewise found that the proportions of large bowel disease diagnosed alone increased most, by 7·6 fold, but combined small and large bowel disease increased by 4·9 fold and small bowel disease alone by 2·2 fold from the first to the third quinquennium of our study. However, re-examination of a sample of earlier records of patients with ulcerative colitis revealed few who could be reclassified as having Crohn's disease. Furthermore, examination of national statistics showed no evidence of a sustained decline in admissions for ulcerative colitis to explain the rise for Crohn's disease in England and Wales generally (Fig. 4.2). The most sensible conclusion would seem to be that some diagnostic reclassification may have occurred, but that the overall rise in

* Calculated from admission rates – see text, and adapted.

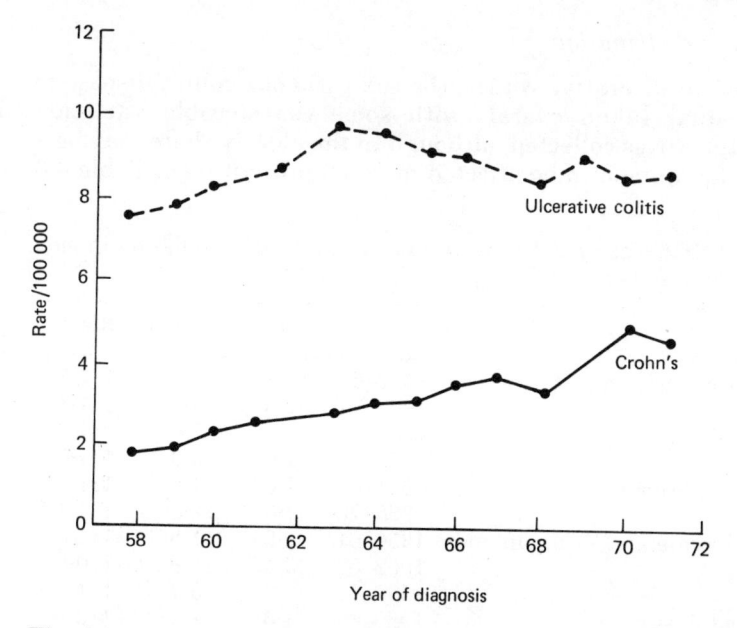

Fig. 4.2 Annual patient discharge rate for Crohn's disease and ulcerative colitis in England and Wales 1958–71*

diagnoses of Crohn's disease in the United Kingdom and in Scandinavia is too great to be attributable entirely to manipulative factors, or to better diagnostic techniques.

Data from hospitals in the USA (Table 4.2) suggest that the number of hospital admissions, and by inference incidence rates, may not be rising, but the time period available for analysis may be too short for any trend to be discernible.

Table 4.2 Time trend in regional enteritis and ulcerative colitis in hospital admissions in 37 selected areas in the USA.[11]

	1969	1971	1973
Regional enteritis			
Observed	274	269	303
Expected	272	283	291
Ratio:	1·01	0·95	1·04
Ulcerative colitis			
Observed	424	403	429
Expected	404	420	431
Ratio:	1·05	0·96	0·99

* Hospital Inpatient Enquiry for England & Wales. Unpublished data, adapted; see text.

Age and sex distribution

In contrast to ulcerative colitis, the sex ratio of Crohn's disease is roughly equal taken overall with some considerable variation between the series collected, although in the elderly there may be a tendency for women to be affected more often than men. Table 4.3

Table 4.3 Crohn's disease. Incidence rates per 100 000 population in men and women.

		Men	Women	Ratio
England, Nottingham	1962–67	1·7	2·2	1:1·3
	1968–72	2·6	3·7	1:1·4
Scotland, Aberdeen[4]	1955–61	1·4	1·6	1:1·1
	1962–68	1·9	3·0	1:1·6
Clydeside[12]	1961–65	1·0	1·6	1:1·6
	1966–70	1·6	2·2	1:1·4
Sweden, Uppsala and Vastmanland[10]	1956–61	1·8	1·8	1:1·0
	1962–67	3·4	2·8	1:0·8
	1968–73	4·3	5·7	1:1·3
Switzerland, Basle[7]	1960–69	1·8	1·4	1:0·8
USA, Baltimore[3]	1960–63	2·5	1·2	1:0·5

Table 4.4 Age and sex distribution of patients at onset of Crohn's disease compared with the general population in Nottingham, England, and in Aberdeen, Scotland.[13]

Age	Men Patients %	Men Controls %	Women Patients %	Women Controls %
Nottingham				
0–19	8·0	32·8	5·8	30·3
20–39	49·0	26·8	48·1	25·9
40–59	24·0	25·2	25·2	24·4
60 or more	20·0	15·2	20·9	19·4
Total number	100	363 882	160	379 201
Aberdeen				
0–19	20·0	34·8	17·9	30·6
20–39	50·0	26·2	36·9	25·0
40–59	15·0	24·8	30·2	25·4
60 or more	15·0	15·2	15·0	19·0
Total number	60	210 000	101	232 000

shows the sex ratios found in some recent series and illustrates these points. Crohn's disease is commonly considered a disease of young adult life, or alternatively to have a peak of incidence then, and a second in old age. Table 4.4 contrasts the proportions of patients of differing ages found in Nottingham and in Aberdeen. It shows that the chances of developing Crohn's disease are about double expectation from the size of the population at risk in young adult life. Thereafter the chances fall, but only to the level to be expected, given the size of the population at risk. However, Crohn's disease in childhood and adolescence is clearly rare when considered on this population basis, as is common clinical experience.

Socio-economic factors No clear social class distribution for Crohn's disease has emerged, nor do people in any specific occupation seem to be at special risk. Table 4.5 shows the occupational

Table 4.5 Socio-economic groups of patients with Crohn's disease and of the general population in Nottingham.[15]

	Percentage of patients	Percentage of population
Managers	13·1	8·4
Professional	4·6	3·0
Intermediate non-manual	3·8	6·8
Junior non-manual	12·7	19·4
Skilled manual	40·0	29·2
Semi-skilled manual	16·9	20·2
Unskilled manual	3·5	6·6
Self-employed	0·8	3·7
Others	4·6	2·7
Total number	260	353 090

groupings of Nottingham patients by broad categories compared with the jobs undertaken by the general population. Minor variations are recorded but consideration of individual jobs does not suggest that more detailed analyses would be helpful. Kyle in Aberdeen likewise found no differences in incidence according to social class,[13] although in Baltimore it seemed that those of higher educational attainment might be affected slightly more often than others.[14] In north-eastern Scotland and in Baltimore town dwellers were affected more often than country dwellers. This difference may at least in part reflect a greater use of medical services by townspeople. However, in Sweden no difference in incidence could be detected between urban and rural residents.[10]

Dietary factors The relative infrequency of Crohn's disease and the unknown, but probably long, incubation period before the disease is clinically manifest and diagnosed hinders any attempts to look for dietary causes. No convincing association with the earlier consumption of specific foods has yet been demonstrated. Suggestions of, for instance, an association for cereal intake[16] are difficult to verify because of the problems of deciding whether patients' views on previous dietary habits are accurate. These have not been confirmed in later data.

Since Crohn's disease is predominantly a western disease in populations with high mobility in habits as well as geographical mobility, the chances of finding a link with any specific dietary item must be low. In addition, reliable figures showing the incidence of Crohn's disease in Western countries are so few even where the disease is well recognized; and the differences in frequency, by contrast with cancer, are so small, that comparisons of affected populations are unlikely to be fruitful. Furthermore, the differences from tropical areas where the disease is rare are so great that no useful information can be gained.

The possibility exists that food additives or changed preservative methods are responsible for the increasing frequency of Crohn's disease, but no additive has so far been shown experimentally to cause Crohn's-like lesions – though certain metals can induce granulomata – and the means by which changed preservative methods could induce disease are unclear.

Possible origins of Crohn's disease

Contagion The clinical contrast between tropical areas where infective diarrhoeas are endemic, and occidental countries where they are less common, has led to the suggestion that non-specific inflammatory bowel disease may represent an unusual response to infection.

Evidence to support a contagion hypothesis is virtually entirely experimental. Extracts of Crohn's disease tissue have been shown by some to cause granulomatous lesions either in injected footpad tissues or within the bowel in mice and rabbits, sometimes producing granulomatous lesions in bowel distant from the sites of injection. In addition the granulomatous lesions or the drainage lymph nodes could be used to pass the lesions into other experimental animals. Control tissues produced no such reaction, and tissue extracts would continue to excite reactions after freezing to $-70°C$, but not after autoclaving.[17-19]

Further evidence, in support of a viral hypothesis, has included the demonstration of cytopathic effects of 220-nanometre tissue filtrates for lung fibroblasts and for rabbit ileal fibroblast cultures, where a 30 nm particle resembling a virus has been found. More recently, 220 nm filtrates of Crohn's disease tissue but not control tissues have been shown to have their cytopathogenic effects inhibited by Nebraska calf-diarrhoea-virus vaccine, confirming the likely presence of reovirus-like particles. The particle size on this occasion was 55–60 nm.[20–22]

By contrast, others have failed to induce granulomatous lesions with Crohn's disease tissue extracts, to demonstrate virus particles by immunoelectron microscopy, or to demonstrate antibody responses to Coxsackie B adenoviruses and EB viruses.[13,23–25]

Further investigation is clearly needed to decide if viral isolates are due to the presence of passenger organisms and to confirm specificity for Crohn's disease inflammatory tissue, but reoviruses are attractive candidates particularly if cross-reactivity with agents known to cause acute diarrhoea can be confirmed.

Epidemiological support for the contagion hypothesis would substantially be derived by showing that people were in the right place at the right time to infect one another. Crohn's disease occurs within families more often than would be expected by chance, but husband and wife pairs with Crohn's disease or with Crohn's disease and ulcerative colitis have scarcely been reported, suggesting a dominance of genetic over environmental influences.

Cold lymphocytotoxic and RNA antibodies have been detected in one study in 40% of patients, 50% of their spouses, 40% of household contacts and 19% of non-household contacts. These results are non-specific but they are compatible with the presence of an environmental viral agent.[26,27]

Deliberate searches for evidence of time–space clustering of Crohn's disease in the Nottingham area have been disappointing. Two different mathematical approaches have been used, one looking at the randomness or otherwise of patient distribution and the other comparing the patterns of distribution of matched patient and control pairs.[28,29] Table 4.6 illustrates the findings in one of these studies and shows no difference in any of the comparisons made between patients and controls for a variety of distances and time intervals. Such studies do not deny absolutely the possibility of contagion, for the degree and manner of contact may be more subtle than even the complex techniques of space–time analysis can detect. However, this, combined with the lack of husband and wife pairs, suggests that simple close contact is unlikely to be related to disease incidence. A combination of a specific genetic constitution with the appropriate environmental circumstances is likely to be needed.

Bacterial infections The presence of sarcoid-like granulomata inevitably suggests an unusual form of mycobacterial infection, but no likely organism has yet been identified. Crohn's disease patients are neither particularly responsive nor anergic in responses to tuberculin, but these findings do not necessarily refute the suggestion that other varieties of mycobacteria are involved, although one

Table 4.6 Analysis of paired persons by workplaces and schools from five years before onset of disease to onset for (a) controls, (b) cases and controls, (c) cases.[29]

Distance between pairs (km)		Up to 1	2–4	5–7	8–10	11–13	14–25	26–37	38–47	48–61
(a) Controls										
0·1	O	70	65	61	54	51	28	21	17	13
	E	71	65	58	52	49	27	16	12	8
0·25	O	167	158	142	126	121	70	49	36	25
	E	176	162	143	127	120	65	42	27	18
0·5	O	421	397	354	332	308	163	118	77	49
	E	443	408	370	336	313	176	124	80	52
1·0	O	1043	989	895	830	780	477	331	202	134
	E	1104	1029	945	857	803	485	348	231	150
(b) Cases and controls										
0·1	O	75	68	57	50	47	26	12	8	4
	E	71	65	58	52	49	27	16	12	8
0·25	O	185	166	145	127	118	60	33	16	12
	E	176	162	143	127	120	65	42	27	18
0·5	O	450	407	368	329	306	180	121	78	51
	E	443	408	370	336	313	176	124	80	52
1·0	O	1127	1041	957	850	793	475	347	238	150
	E	1104	1029	945	857	803	485	348	231	150
(c) Cases										
0·1	O	15	14	13	13	12	6	3	3	2
	E	18	16	15	13	12	7	4	3	2
0·25	O	45	40	35	33	31	17	13	8	4
	E	44	40	36	32	30	16	11	7	5
0·5	O	126	114	110	95	91	54	40	26	16
	E	111	102	92	84	78	44	31	20	13
1·0	O	315	287	274	249	233	139	106	80	54
	E	276	257	236	214	201	121	87	58	38

Period of time at specified distance (months)

O = Observed number of pairs; E = Expected number of pairs.

study failed to demonstrate sensitivity to atypical mycobacterial antigens.[30] The analogy with sarcoidosis extends to the presence of positive Kveim reactions in at least some patients with Crohn's disease,[31] but the clinical characteristics of the diseases and their epidemiological features are disparate. Recently evidence has been adduced to suggest that cell wall-deficient variants of mycobacteria and pseudomonas species may be of aetiological importance,[72,73] no epidemiological support is available. Yersinial acute ileitis does not predispose to Crohn's disease.[32]

Ulcerative colitis

The diagnostic spectrum of ulcerative colitis runs from limited proctitis to inflammatory disease which extends throughout the large intestine. Clinically epidemiologically there are no distinctive features about patients with greater or lesser amounts of disease, and those who present initially with proctitis may or may not go on to develop extensive colitis; others present with severe life-threatening disease. Because of this clinical range and because the proportions of individuals with mild and severe disease are unknown, measurement of incidence and prevalence rates is difficult. Mortality rates are clearly unsatisfactory, since only a minor proportion of patients die, and deaths are at least as likely to be due to secondary disease, such as pneumonia as a post-operative complication, as to the colitis itself. Hospital admission rates are also difficult to relate to disease incidence rates, because patients with mild disease may never be admitted.

The diagnosis of ulcerative colitis itself can usually be made with confidence at least in western countries, where infective dysenteries are rare, because the rectum is always involved in colitis and it is therefore possible to see the abnormality sigmoidoscopically. Other varieties of non-infective colitis such as ischaemic disease are probably so rare that mistaken inclusion as non-specific ulcerative colitis poses no problems in numerical terms. Crohn's disease of the colon presents more difficulty because the distinction between granulomatous disease, which is usually segmental and tends to spare the rectum, from classical ulcerative colitis is not as clear as might initially appear.

Incidence and time trends

Incidence Table 4.7 shows the average annual incidence and prevalence rates recorded for ulcerative colitis in seven surveys. The figures are reasonably consistent with each other, the lowest figure being recorded in Norway which also showed the lowest incidence rate for Crohn's disease. All the figures are likely to be underestimated because patients with mild inflammatory disease are probably under-recorded. They are seldom admitted to hospital and no comprehensive system of recording out-patient attendances has yet been devised. Experience in Nottingham suggests that at least as many patients with mild ulcerative colitis never needing admission attend for consultation as are admitted with more severe disease.

Estimates of disease frequency from other areas are little more than guesses. The prevalence of colitis is probably low in most tropical areas and in the southern part of Europe, but the extent to which incidence figures are obscured by the high frequency of infective bowel disease is unknown. In New Zealand though colitis

Table 4.7 Ulcerative colitis. Average annual incidence rates or first hospital admission rates and prevalence rates per 100 000 population.

		Incidence	Prevalence
Denmark, Copenhagen[33]	1961–66	7·3	44·1
England, Oxford[2]	1951–60	6·5	79·9
Israel, Tel Aviv[34]	1961–70	3·6	37·4
New Zealand, Wellington[35]	1954–58	5·6	41·3
Norway, general survey[6]	1956–60	2·3	
	1964–69	3·3	
USA, Baltimore[3]	1960–63	4·6	42·0
Minnesota*[36]	1935–44	4·4	
	1945–54	7·4	
	1955–64	8·7	88·0 (in 1965)

* Excludes transient proctitis and discontinuous disease.

was recorded as commonly as in Northern Europe in people of European extraction, it was very rarely found in Maoris,[35] — the reasons are unclear. Descriptions of groups of cases, which are often large, have been reported from Eastern Europe (Czechoslovakia),[37] Greece,[38] Turkey,[39] Japan[40] and India,[41,42] amongst others, but the prevalence or incidence of the disease compared with Northern Europe is impossible to gauge. Seven-fold differences in hospital admission rates in India (between Bombay and Ahmedabad) have been recorded,[41] which suggest that there may be pronounced regional variation.

Time trends The detection of chronological changes in incidence rates is hampered by a number of factors. These include difficulty in ensuring that disease of equivalent severity is being detected in different time periods, since estimates of incidence depend primarily on the measurement of hospital admission, and the problems of allowing for diagnostic transfer from colitis to Crohn's disease with the growing acceptance of the clinical entity of Crohn's disease of the colon.

Hospital admission data in the United Kingdom suggest that, though fluctuations have occurred, ulcerative colitis has become no more frequent a cause of admission as time has passed (Fig. 4.2). However, the diagnosis of ulcerative colitis has become more common in some epidemiological series, though the change is not so pronounced as for Crohn's disease. In Minnesota, USA[36] diagnoses of proctitis and ulcerative colitis became more common from 1935 to 1965 (Table 4.7), and in Scandinavia a rising incidence has been recorded in Norway from 1956 to 1969,[6] but not in Sweden.[10] The meaning of such trends is hard to establish. Though in areas such as England and Sweden where Crohn's disease has become prevalent, the diagnosis of ulcerative colitis does not seem to have been made any more or less frequently as time has passed; in Norway both diagnoses have become more common. Disentangling the various and often contradictory effects of changing admission policies for inflammatory bowel disease, changing fashions in diagnostic labels, and (probably) increasing diagnostic likelihood through greater awareness and better methods of investigation makes any firm judgements about changes in the frequency of ulcerative colitis impossible.

Age and sex incidence

Ulcerative colitis is generally considered to be more prevalent in women than in men, and to have its onset most frequently in early adult life. Table 4.8 gives the proportions of women recorded in four

Table 4.8 Ulcerative colitis: overall incidence rates per 100 000 population in men and women.

		Men	Women	Ratio
Denmark, Copenhagen[33]	1961–66	6·7	7·6	1:1·1
England, Oxford[2]	1951–60	5·8	7·3	1:1·3
Norway, general survey[43]	1956–60	2·0	2·1	1:1·1
USA, Baltimore[3]	1960–63	3·9	5·2	1:1·3

different epidemiological surveys. Women were found to be affected more often than men in all of these, but the differences were not great.

Examination of age incidence patterns has confirmed that colitis has its peak incidence in early adult life (Table 4.9), but diagnoses continue to be made throughout life. A secondary peak of incidence has been claimed in the elderly, partially based upon the figures from Oxford given in this table. Hardly any such trend is detectable in the data from Norway and from Copenhagen, except in men. If there is a secondary peak in the elderly, and the supporting evidence is poor, then it has been proposed that it could represent a different type of disease, associated with ischaemia. Clinical and pathological evidence to support this view is lacking, basically because there are no useful discriminants which allow ischaemic disease to be identified confidently. Atherosclerotic changes in abdominal vessels are common in the presence or absence of colonic disease, large vessel occlusion is seldom detectable arteriographically in those with 'typical' segmental ischaemic colitis, and there are no characteristic histological abnormalities.

Table 4.9 Ulcerative colitis. Average annual incidence rates by age and sex.

Oxford, 1951–60[2]			Norway, 1964–69[6]		Copenhagen, 1961–66[33]	
Age	Men	Women	Age	Both sexes	Men	Women
0–14	0·6	1·3	0–9	0·3	0·4	1·4
15–24	4·7	4·0	10–19	1·6	6·2	4·6
25–34	8·2	10·9	20–29	5·8	11·6	12·3
35–44	9·2	12·1	30–39	4·8	12·4	8·2
45–54	8·2	8·6	40–49	4·3	7·0	7·9
55–64	7·6	8·8	50–59	3·8	10·3	7·5
65–74	8·7	12·7	60–69	2·9	6·7	7·8
75+	2·5	5·7	70–79	1·8	8·4	0
			80+	1·5	0	13·9*

* Small numbers.

Environmental factors

Socio-economic factors Any differences in socio-economic status of patients with ulcerative colitis from the pattern seen in control populations are likely to be small. A tendency towards a greater incidence of colitis in the relatively well-off has been noted in Denmark,[44] but no such difference was detectable in the USA or elsewhere.

Patients with ulcerative colitis are commonly believed to have been subject to psychological pressures which predisposed to the occurrence of their disease. Supporting evidence for this concept is limited, basically because it is hard to find out about the psychological make-up and reaction of patients prior to disease onset. Comparison of illness experience and stress factors in patients with ulcerative colitis and the irritable bowel syndrome in Baltimore showed that those with the irritable bowel were, if anything, more likely to have had severe illness or to be exposed to psychological stresses than those with colitis.[45,46]

Dietary factors No sound evidence is available to associate the occurrence of ulcerative colitis with any dietary habit or pattern. The pathological features of the disease with mucosal lymphoid and plasma cell infiltration, and the demonstration of antibodies to colonic mucosa which cross-react with specific serotypes of *Escherichia coli*, suggest that an altered bacterial flora, perhaps secondary to dietary factors, may be important in the genesis of the disease. The description of patients with milk intolerance led to the hypothesis that milk sensitivity might be important, perhaps induced by early weaning. However, later work makes it more likely that milk intolerance is due to an incapacity in some patients of the small bowel mucosa to break down milk sugar.

High titres of circulating antibodies to cow's milk proteins have been found more frequently in patients with ulcerative colitis than in healthy controls.[47] However, antibody titres were not related to the severity of the disease, nor were they affected by milk withdrawal. Later no differences were detected in antibody titres in colitics and controls,[48] and skin tests for reaginic antibodies failed to show any differences between patients with colitis, Crohn's disease and the irritable bowel syndrome or normal controls (Table 4.10).[49]

Table 4.10 Frequency of positive skin tests to milk proteins.[49]

	Number tested	Casein	a-Lactalbumin	β-Lactoglobulin
Ulcerative colitis	39	59	10	13
Crohn's disease	19	68	21	12
Normal individuals and irritable bowel syndrome	39	72	18	18

Over-refining of carbohydrate foods has been advanced as another important predisposing factor. Virtually the only evidence to support this view is the suggestion that bowel cancer in the absence of colitis, and colitis itself, may share common geographical patterns of incidence. This subject is discussed in more detail on p. 65.

Infection and colitis induction

Although the distinction between infective dysenteries and ulcerative colitis was made over a hundred years ago by Samuel Wilks,[50] a relationship to the infective condition was accepted. This was largely supported by the isolation of dysenteric organisms from the faeces of some patients with chronic colitis, by the apparent response of some patients to polyvalent antidysenteric sera, and by the finding of high agglutination titres to *Shigella* in the sera of patients with colitis.[51,52] Such observations have not been confirmed since, but altered immunological reactivity has been demonstrated in colitic patients. The *in vitro* migration of leucocytes obtained from patients can be inhibited by colonic mucosal extracts: lymphocytes of colitics have cytotoxic activity for colonic epithelial cells, and haemagglutinating antibodies can be demonstrated to colonic epithelial tissue.[53-55] To add to these observations, cross-reactivity can be shown between anticolon antibodies and the lipopolysaccharide antigen of *E. coli* 014, and lymphocytotoxicity for colonic epithelial cells can be inhibited by prior incubation of the patient's lymphocytes with a lipopolysaccharide extract of *E. coli* 0119.B14.[56,57]

These observations suggest that ulcerative colitis could be caused by an alteration of immune processes with disturbance of immune recognition of intestinal mucosa and colonic bacteria. Epidemiological evidence to support such a hypothesis is weak and fragmentary. The probable inverse geographical correlation of the incidence of infective dysenteries and ulcerative colitis is one such piece of evidence. Patients with colitis have also been shown by some to have an alteration in the bacterial flora of the bowel with increased numbers of coliform organisms,[58] though whether observations on bacterial flora after the onset of disease can be transposed to relate to conditions prior to and initiating the onset of disease must be extremely doubtful. The geographical distribution of *E. coli* serotypes and the distribution of ulcerative colitis have never been compared, nor is there any evidence about accessory environmental factors which might predispose to colitis and alter *E. coli* or other bacterial populations in the bowel.

Factors in common to colitis and Crohn's disease

Associated diseases

Inflammatory disease   A group of non-specific conditions, including large joint arthritis, uveitis, ankylosing spondylitis and chronic active liver disease occur in association with ulcerative colitis and Crohn's disease. No obvious epidemiological morals can be discerned in these associations which seem likely to be due to the participance of a common pathogenic mechanism, perhaps through altered immunological reactivity. An increase in the proportions of patients with urticaria, asthma and allergic rhinitis supports this possibility in ulcerative colitis.[59]

Gallstones   Patients who have had ileal resections appear to be unduly prone to gallstones due to a reduced bile salt pool through failure of ileal reabsorption of bile acids. The increase in stone frequency is perceptible, but not dramatic when compared with the high general population incidence of gallstones. The association of gallstones with Crohn's disease therefore reflects a consequence of Crohn's disease and not a second independent action of an aetiological agent.

Peptic ulcer Suggestions that ulcer incidence is increased in patients with inflammatory bowel disease are ill-founded.

Cancer Associations have been found between liability to large bowel cancer in ulcerative colitis, and to small and large bowel cancer in Crohn's disease.[60,61] One instance of small intestinal cancer was noted in 449 patients with Crohn's disease in the USA[62] and we have noted a single case in our series of four hundred patients with Crohn's disease. These instances have to be taken in conjunction with further case reports, and compared with the very low frequency of cancer of the small intestine in the general population. In Crohn's disease the overall risk of colonic cancer is again low; eight instances were noted in a group of 356 patients with colonic inflammatory disease, none occurring in a remaining group of 93 patients with small bowel inflammation only.[61] By comparison with the general population colorectal cancer was twenty times as common as would have been expected by chance, but this still represents a small figure.

The risk of cancer in the colon in ulcerative colitis is virtually confined to patients whose inflammatory disease has spread proximal to the splenic flexure and who have had colitic symptoms for at least ten years (Tables 4.11 and 4.12).[63,64] Patients with childhood onset of colitis are generally considered to have a particular risk of cancer supervening, but this may simply be due to the large time

Table 4.11 The risk of cancer in ulcerative colitis: influence of disease extent.[63]

	Number of cases of colitis	Patient years of follow-up	Number of cases of cancer
No radiological change	132	1005	0
Distal disease	291	1952	1
Disease present proximal to splenic flexure	196	1156	9

Table 4.12 The risk of cancer in ulcerative colitis: influence of disease duration in patients with extensive disease only.[64]

Duration of symptoms in years	Number of cases of colitis	Percentage annual incidence of cancer
1–9	151	0·4
10–19	33	2·0
20+	26	5·8

period available for cancer to develop. The distribution of cancer in the large bowel tends to be more proximal than in cancer without colitis, but the reasons are unclear. Bile duct tumours have also been recorded occasionally in ulcerative colitis. The reasons are again unclear. As such tumours are ordinarily rare the association is likely to be real, and might perhaps be related to another association between sclerosing cholangitis and ulcerative colitis.

Ethnic variation

In the United States both ulcerative colitis and Crohn's disease have been detected less frequently in the black and Indian populations than in whites. In Baltimore black people were about one-third as likely to be affected by ulcerative colitis and one-fifth as likely to develop Crohn's disease as the whites. This difference is reflected in mortality rates (Table 4.13). No logical reasons for such variations

Table 4.13 Crude death rates per 100 000 population for chronic enteritis and colitis according to race and sex: United States 1959–61.[65]

	Total	Men	Women
White	1·9	1·7	2·0
Non-white	1·0	0·9	1·0
Negro	1·0	0·9	1·0
Indian	1·0	1·0	1·0
Chinese	1·0	1·5	0·3
Japanese	0·8	1·2	0·5
Other	0·6	0·9	0·2

are detectable. Poor access to hospital facilities might explain some of the differences, but not in the Baltimore population where general access is said to be good. In general, genetically determined resistance to the development of the disease seems less likely than a reduced prevalence of predisposing environmental factors.

A greater prevalence of ulcerative colitis in Jews than in non-Jews has been recorded in United States veterans (Table 4.14), and

Table 4.14 Proportions of Jews with ulcerative colitis and Crohn's disease amongst United States veterans admitted to hospital.[66]

	Number of Jews	Total patients (all white)	Percentage Jews
Crohn's disease	65	698	9·3
Ulcerative colitis	111	1129	9·8
Sample of general medical and surgical discharges	80	3469	2·3

in the population of Baltimore. No such increase seems to have been detected elsewhere except in an early study in London. The epidemiological moral of a greater prevalence in Jews is uncertain. In Israel itself the prevalence of colitis has been found to be greater in people born in Europe or America than in Asia or Africa (Table 4.15).

Table 4.15 Age standardized prevalence rates of ulcerative colitis in Jews in Tel Aviv according to place of birth.[34]

Birthplace	Total cases	Population	Prevalence* per 100 000
Israel	31	165 854	25·8
Asia	12	49 870	18·9
Africa	6	20 316	18·5
Europe and America	74	143 808	37·3

Genetic factors

Crohn's disease and ulcerative colitis each occurs more commonly within families than would be expected by chance, and those same families have an increased frequency of the other disease.[67,68] Table 4.16 illustrates this finding: it also shows that the overall chances of

Table 4.16 Relationships of inflammatory bowel disease patients in Liverpool.[67]

	Ulcerative colitis (UC)	Crohn's disease (CD)
Propositi	103	39
First degree relatives with UC	4	4
First degree relatives with CD	3	7
Second degree relatives with UC	1	1
Second degree relatives with CD	1	1

a second family member developing Crohn's disease, or ulcerative colitis are low, though given the much lower prevalence of the diseases generally in the population there is still a clear rise. Two affected siblings tends to be the commonest pattern, followed by parent and child and then second or third degree relatives.

The basis for the familial incidence is unclear, common environmental factors may in part explain the occurrences, but the paucity

* Standardized rates.

of reports of husband and wife pairs suggests that such influences might operate earlier rather than later in life, unless the requirement is a combination of specific constitutional and environmental factors.

Genetic associations Specific factors which have been examined include the ABO blood groups, secretor status,[69] and glucose-6-phosphate dehydrogenase deficiency. No associations were detected. Examination for possible associations within the HLA system have yielded conflicting reports and taken overall, no association seems likely.[67,70,71] The associations between HLA B27 and ankylosing spondylitis and between ankylosing spondylitis and inflammatory bowel disease have been examined together. There is a suggestion that those who have Crohn's disease and HLA-B27 are much more likely to have ankylosing spondylitis than if they were HLA-B27 alone, but that the possession of HLA-B27 does not increase the likelihood of Crohn's disease or ulcerative colitis themselves.[67]

References

1. Lockhart Mummery, H. E., Morson, B. C. (1960). Crohn's disease (regional enteritis) of the large intestine and its distinction from ulcerative colitis. *Gut* **1**, 87–105.
2. Evans, J. G., Acheson, E. D. (1965). An epidemiological study of ulcerative colitis and regional enteritis in the Oxford area. *Gut* **6**, 311–24.
3. Monk, M., Mendeloff, A. I., Siegel, C. I., Lilienfeld, A. (1967). An epidemiological study of ulcerative colitis and regional enteritis among adults in Baltimore. I, Hospital incidence and prevalence, 1960–63. *Gastroenterology* **53**, 198–210.
4. Kyle, J. (1971). An epidemiological study of Crohn's disease in North East Scotland. *Gastroenterology* **61**, 826–33.
5. Miller, D. S., Keighley, A. C., Langman, M. J. S. (1974). Changing patterns in epidemiology of Crohn's disease. *Lancet* **2**, 691–3.
6. Myren, J., Gjone, E., Hertzberg, J. N., Rygvold, O., Semb, L. S., Fretheim, B. (1971). Epidemiology of Ulcerative Colitis and Regional Enteritis (Crohn's Disease) in Norway. *Scandinavian Journal of Gastroenterology* **6**, 511–14.
7. Fahrländer, H., Baerlocher, C. (1970). Epidemiology of Crohn's disease in the Basle area. In *Regional Enteritis. Crohn's Disease. Fifth Skandia International Symposium*, ed. Engel, A., Larssen, T. Stockholm, Nordiska Bokhandelus Forlag.
8. Höj, L., Brix-Jensen, P., Bonnevie, O., Riis, P. (1973). An epidemiological study of regional enteritis in Copenhagen County and Gentofte municipality. *Scandinavian Journal of Gastroenterology* **8**, 381–4.
9. Wenckert, A., Henriksson, A., Lindström, C. (1974). Incidence of Crohn's disease in the city of Malmö. *Scandinavian Journal of Gastroenterology* **9**, suppl. 27, 42.

10. Bergman, L., Krause, U. (1975). The incidence of Crohn's disease in central Sweden. *Scandinavian Journal of Gastroenterology* **10,** 725–9.
11. Kaplan, S. D. (1975). Time trend in regional enteritis. *Professional Activity Study Reporter* **14,** No. 9, 1–5.
12. Smith, I. S., Young, S., Gillespie, G., O'Connor, J., Bell, J. R. (1975). Epidemiological aspects of Crohn's disease in Clydesdale, 1961–70. *Gut* **16,** 62–7.
13. Kyle, J. (1972). *Crohn's Disease.* London, Heinemann.
14. Monk, M., Mendeloff, A. I., Siegel, C. I., Lilienfeld, A. (1969). An epidemiological study of ulcerative colitis and regional enteritis among adults in Baltimore. II, Social and demographic factors. *Gastroenterology* **56,** 847–57.
15. Keighley, A., Miller, D. S., Hughes, A. O., Langman, M. J. S. (1976). The demographic and social characteristics of patients with Crohn's disease in the Nottingham area. *Scandinavian Journal of Gastroenterology* **11,** 293–6.
16. James, A. H. (1977). Breakfast and Crohn's disease. *British Medical Journal* **1,** 943–5.
17. Mitchell, D. N., Rees, R. J. W. (1969). Agent transmissible from Crohn's disease tissue. *Lancet* **2,** 168–71.
18. Cave, D. R., Mitchell, D. N., Brooke, B. N. (1976). Evidence of an agent transmissible from ulcerative colitis tissue. *Lancet* **1,** 1311–14.
19. Cave, D. R., Mitchell, D. N., Kane, S. P., Brooke, B. N. (1973). Further animal evidence of a transmissible agent in Crohn's disease. *Lancet* **2,** 1120–2.
20. Gitnick, G. L., Rosen, V. I. (1976). Electron microscopic studies of viral agents in Crohn's disease. *Lancet* **2,** 217–19.
21. Gitnick, G. L., Arthur, M. H., Shibata, I. (1976). Cultivation of viral agents from Crohn's disease. *Lancet* **2,** 215–17.
22. Whorwell, P. J., Phillips, C. A., Beeken, W. L., Little, P. K., Roessner, K. D. (1977). Isolation of reovirus-like agents from patients with Crohn's disease. *Lancet* **1,** 1169–71.
23. Bolton, P. M., Owen, E., Heatley, R. V., Williams, W. J., Hughes, L. E. (1973). Negative findings in laboratory animals for a transmissible agent in Crohn's disease. *Lancet* **2,** 1122–4.
24. Jarnerot, G., Lantorp, K. (1972). Antibodies to E.B. virus in cases of Crohn's disease. *New England Journal of Medicine* **286,** 1215–16.
25. Whorwell, P. J., Baldwin, R. C., Wright, R. (1976). Ferritin in Crohn's disease tissue: detection by electron microscopy. *Gut* **17,** 696–9.
26. Korsmeyer, S., Strickland, R. G., Wilson, I. D., Williams, R. C. Jr. (1974). Serum lymphocytotoxic and lymphocytophilic antibody activity in inflammatory bowel disease. *Gastroenterology* **67,** 578–83.
27. Korsmeyer, S. J., Williams, R. C., Wilson, I. D., Strickland, R. G. (1975). Lymphocytotoxic antibody in inflammatory bowel disease: a family study. *New England Journal of Medicine* **293,** 1117–20.
28. Miller, D. S., Keighley, A., Smith, P. G., Hughes, A. O., Langman, M. J. S. (1975). Crohn's disease in Nottingham: a search for time–space clustering. *Gut* **16,** 454–7.
29. Miller, D. S., Keighley, A., Smith, P. G., Hughes, A. O., Langman, M. J. S. (1976). A case-control method for seeking evidence of contagion in Crohn's disease. *Gastroenterology* **71,** 385–7.
30. Morganroth, J., Watson, D. W. (1970). Sensitivity to atypical mycobac-

terial antigens in patients with Crohn's disease. *American Journal of Digestive Diseases* **15**, 653–6.
31. Mitchell, D. N., Cannon, P., Dyer, N. H., Hinson, K. F. W., Willoughby, J. M. T. (1969). The Kveim, test in Crohn's disease. *Lancet* **2**, 571–3.
32. Sjöström, B. (1971). Acute terminal ileitis and its relation to Crohn's disease. In *Regional Enteritis. Crohn's Disease. Fifth Skandia International Symposium*, ed. Engel, A., Larssen, T. Stockholm, Nordiska Bokhandelus Forlag.
33. Bonnevie, O., Riis, P., Anthonisen, P. (1968). An epidemiological study of ulcerative colitis in Copenhagen County. *Scandinavian Journal of Gastroenterology* **3**, 432–8.
34. Gilat, T., Ribak, J., Benaroya, Y., Zemishlany, Z., Weissman, I. (1974). Ulcerative colitis in the Jewish population of Tel-Aviv Jafo. *Gastroenterology* **66**, 335–42.
35. Wigley, R. D., MacLaurin, B. P. (1962). A study of ulcerative colitis in New Zealand, showing a low incidence in Maoris. *British Medical Journal* **2**, 228–31.
36. Sedlack, R. E., Nobrega, F. T., Kurland, L. T., Sauer, W. G. (1972). Inflammatory colon disease in Rochester, Minnesota, 1935–1964. *Gastroenterology* **62**, 935–41.
37. Nedbal, J., Maratka, Z. (1968). Ulcerative procto-colitis in Czechoslovakia. *American Journal of Proctology* **19**, 106–13.
38. Zevgolatis, C., Economopoulos, P., Sakellaropoulos, N. (1969). Ulcerative colitis in Greece. A study of 181 cases. *Proceedings of the Royal Society of Medicine* **62**, 261.
39. Aktan, H., Paykoc, Z., Erian, A. (1970). Ulcerative colitis in Turkey: clinical review of sixty cases. *Diseases of the colon and rectum* **13**, 62–6.
40. Matsunaga, F. (1959). Clinical studies on ulcerative colitis and its related diseases in Japan. In *Proceedings of the World Congress of Gastroenterology, Washington, 1958*, vol. 2, 955–60. Baltimore, Williams and Wilkins.
41. Chuttani, H. K., Nigam, S. P., Sarna, S. K., Dhanda, P. C., Gupta, P. S. (1967). Ulcerative colitis in the tropics. *British Medical Journal* **4**, 204–7.
42. Tandon, B. N., Mathur, A. K., Mohapatra, L. N., Tandon, H. N., Wig, K. L. (1965). A study of the prevalence and clinical pattern of non-specific ulcerative colitis in northern India. *Gut* **6**, 448–53.
43. Gjone, E., Myren, J. (1964). Colitis ulcerosa i Norge. *Nordisk Medicin* **71**, 143–5.
44. Bonnevie, O. (1967). A socio-economic study of patients with ulcerative colitis. *Scandinavian Journal of Gastroenterology* **2**, 129–36.
45. Monk, M., Mendeloff, A. I., Siegel, C. I., Lilienfeld, A. (1970). An epidemiological study of ulcerative colitis and regional enteritis among adults in Baltimore. III, Psychological and possible stress-precipitating factors. *Journal of chronic disease* **22**, 565–78.
46. Mendeloff, A. I., Monk, M., Siegel, C. I., Lilienfeld, A. (1970). Illness experience and life stresses in patients with irritable colon and with ulcerative colitis. *New England Journal of Medicine* **282**, 14–17.
47. Taylor, K. B., Truelove, S. C., Wright, R. (1964). Serologic reactions to gluten and cow's proteins in gastro-intestinal disease. *Gastroenterology* **46**, 99–108.
48. Dudek, B., Spiro, H. M., Thayer, W. R. (1965). A study of ulcerative

colitis and circulating antibodies to milk proteins. *Gastroenterology* **49**, 544–7.
49. Jewell, D. P., Truelove, S. C. (1972). Reaginic hypersensitivity in ulcerative colitis. *Gut* **13**, 903–6.
50. Wilks, S. (1859). *Lectures on Pathological Anatomy*. London, Longman, Brown, Green, Longmans and Roberts.
51. Hurst, A. F. (1935). Ulcerative colitis. *Guy's Hospital Reports* **85**, 317–55.
52. Manson Bahr, P. (1943). *The Dysenteric Disorders*. London, Cassell.
53. Bendixen, G. (1969). Cellular hypersensitivity to components of intestinal mucosa in ulcerative colitis and Crohn's disease. *Gut* **10**, 631–6.
54. Perlman, P., Broberger, O. (1963). *In vitro* studies of ulcerative colitis. II, Cytotoxic action of white blood cells from patients on human fetal colon cells. *Journal of Experimental Medicine* **117**, 717–33.
55. Watson, D. W., Quigley, A., Bolt, R. J. (1966). The cytotoxicity of circulating lymphocytes from ulcerative colitis patients for human colon epithelial cells. *Gastroenterology* **50**, 886–7.
56. Lagercrantz, R., Hammarstrom, S., Perlman, P., Gustafsson, B. E. (1966). Immunological studies in ulcerative colitis. IV, Origin of autoantibodies. *Journal of Experimental Medicine* **128**, 1339–52.
57. Shorter, R. G., Cardoza, M. R., Remine, S. G., Spencer, R. J., Huizenga, K. A. (1970). Modification of *in vitro* cytotoxicity of lymphocytes from patients with chronic ulcerative colitis or granulomatous colitis for allogenic colonic epithelial cells. *Gastroenterology* **58**, 692–8.
58. Gorbach, S. L., Nahas, L., Plant, A. G., Weinstein, L., Patterson, J. F., Levitan, R. (1968). Studies of intestinal microflora v. faecal microbial ecology in ulcerative colitis and regional enteritis. *Gastroenterology* **54**, 575–87.
59. Hammer, B., Ashurst, P., Naish, J. (1968). Diseases associated with ulcerative colitis and Crohn's disease. *Gut* **9**, 17–21.
60. Perrett, A. D., Truelove, S. C., Massarella, G. R. (1968). Crohn's disease and carcinoma of the colon. *British Medical Journal* **2**, 466–8.
61. Fielding, J. F., Prior, P., Waterhouse, J. A., Cooke, W. T. (1972). Malignancy in Crohn's disease. *Scandinavian Journal of Gastroenterology* **7**, 3–7.
62. Weedon, D. D., Shorter, R. G., Ilstrup, D. M., Huizenga, K. A., Taylor, W. F. (1973). Crohn's disease and cancer. *New England Journal of Medicine* **289**, 1099–103.
63. MacDougall, I. P. M. (1961). The cancer risk in ulcerative colitis. *Lancet* **2**, 655–8.
64. Watts, J. McK., de Dombal, F. T., Watkinson, G., Goligher, J. C. (1966). Local complications of ulcerative colitis: stricture pseudopolyposis and carcinoma of colon and rectum. *British Medical Journal* **1**, 1442–7.
65. Mendeloff, A. I., Dunn, J. P. (1971). *Digestive Diseases. Vital and Health Statistics Monographs*. American Public Health Association. Cambridge, Mass., Harvard University Press.
66. Acheson, E. D. (1960). The distribution of ulcerative colitis and regional enteritis in United States veterans with particular reference to the Jewish religion. *Gut* **1**, 291–3.
67. Lewkonia, R. M., McConnell, R. B. (1976). Familial inflammatory bowel disease – heredity or environment. *Gut* **17**, 235–43.
68. Binder, V., Weeke, E., Olsen, J. H., Anthonisen, D., Riis, P. (1966). A

genetic study of ulcerative colitis. *Scandinavian Journal of Gastroenterology* **1**, 49–56.
69. Winstone, N. E., Henderson, A. J., Brooke, B. N. (1960). Blood-groups and secretor status in ulcerative colitis. *Lancet* **2**, 64–5.
70. Asquith, P., Mackintosh, P., Stokes, P. L., Holmes, G. K. T., Cooke, W. T. (1974). Histocompatibility antigens in patients with inflammatory bowel disease. *Lancet* **1**, 113–15.
71. Leukonia, R. M., Woodrow, J. C., McConnell, R. B., Evans, D. A. P. (1974). HL-A antigens in inflammatory bowel disease. *Lancet* **1**, 574–5.
72. Burnham, W. R., Lennard Jones, J. E., Stanford, J. L., Bird, R. G. (1978) Mycobacteria as a possible cause of inflammatory bowel disease. *Lancet* **2**, 693–696.
73. Parent, K., Mitchell, P. D. (1978) Cell wall-defective variants of pseudomonas-like (Group Va) bacteria in Crohn's disease. *Gastroenterology*, **75**, 368–372.

5
Diverticular disease and appendicitis

Diverticular disease

Though diverticulosis of the colon is a common finding at barium enema examinations and at post mortem in western countries, there is little reliable information about its epidemiological features.

Whereas 10% or more of the elderly of the population may have colonic diverticula, the clinical patterns of illness associated with them are extremely variable. A minority of patients present with bleeding, perforation or abscess formation. Many will be seen with complaints of variable bowel habit and barium enema examination will be arranged primarily to ensure that no cancer is present. Finally, an unknown proportion will never present with symptoms at all.

Death due to diverticular disease is rare, and virtually unknown before the age of 45.[1] Since death is so infrequent, and essentially is due to complications, the use of death rates to analyse the frequency distribution for all diverticular disease for epidemiological purposes could be dangerously misleading.

Data obtained from clinical series will be more reliable as indicators of disease frequency in the population, but the findings must be determined in part by patterns of referral according to symptoms before radiological examination. Thus, if the prime reason for arranging for barium enema examination is to exclude cancer, then the frequency with which diverticular disease is detected will depend partly upon the degree to which the symptom patterns of diverticular disease and cancer overlap, and partly upon the strength of the clinician's desire to exclude the presence of cancer.

Autopsy series can theoretically provide more reliable data, but suffer from the same defects as do autopsy data about peptic ulcer frequency. The figures will be determined in part by the care with which the colon is examined, and since death is likely to be due to extra-abdominal disease there may be little to induce the pathologist to clean and examine the colon properly. Furthermore, the findings at death in people of differing age groups cannot necessarily be thought to apply to those who remain alive. A six-fold increase in the frequency of recording of the presence of diverticula over a successive series of 7000 post mortem examinations in Australia has been in great part attributed to more careful scrutiny of the bowel.[2]

Incidence, geographical frequency and time trends

Age and sex distribution Colonic diverticula are detected increasingly frequently in white populations with advancing age, and in general no difference has been detectable in this pattern in men and women. Tables 5.1–5.3 show that these trends have been demonstrable in normal volunteers, at necropsy, and at barium enema examination of patients with bowel symptoms.

Table 5.1 Diverticula in volunteers examined by barium follow-through X-ray in Oxford, England.[3]

Age	Men Number examined	Number with diverticula	Women Number examined	Number with diverticula
Less than 40	14	0	25	0
40–59	14	2	13	3
60–79	10	3	14	4
80+	10	3	9	5
Total	48	8	61	12

Table 5.2 Diverticula found at necropsy in Melbourne, Australia.[4]

Age	Number examined	Percentage frequency of diverticula Men	Women
10–30	4	0	0
31–50	23	12	6
51–70	72	41	36
71+	101	54	56

Table 5.3 Annual incidence rates of diverticular disease in Edinburgh, Scotland, 1970–73.[5]

Age	Men	Women
15–44	0·2	0·2
45–59	1·4	1·3
60–74	4·0	3·8
75+	6·2	5·6

Geographical frequency Despite the difficulties of collecting data which give accurate measures of the presence of colonic diverticula, there is good reason for believing that the frequency varies greatly from place to place. Painter has detailed evidence which suggests that diverticula have been rarely detected either at barium enema examination or at post-mortem in the Far East, India, the Middle East and tropical Africa.[6] In all such areas diverticulosis was detected in less than one in a thousand examinations. The figures have been so low, and the agreement so general, that it is very unlikely that the trends are explainable either by systematic under-reporting or by the relative deficiency of elderly people, who are more prone to have diverticular disease.

By contrast, diverticula have been commonly detected in Western European, North American and Australasian populations. Comparison of frequencies between different areas is virtually impossible because of the combined problems of weighting data according to the age structure of the populations examined, taking account of differences which could arise in the care of colonic examination and, in clinical series, of assuring that the indications for examination were similar. Köhler[7] concluded from comparative autopsy studies that, age for age, diverticula were present three times as commonly in inhabitants of South Sweden as in those of Finland (Table 5.4),

Table 5.4 Percentage frequencies of diverticular disease at autopsy in Helsinki, Finland and Lund, Sweden, 1967–68.[7]

Age	Finland	Sweden
21–30	0	1
31–40	2	3
41–50	2	9
51–60	6	18
61–70	8	33
71–80	23	37
81+	19	45

but a barium enema survey conducted some ten years later showed that diverticula were detectable twice as commonly in Finland as in the earlier survey.[8]

Hospital admission statistics are likely to be open to wider errors of interpretation than unselected barium enema or autopsy studies, because a minority of patients have sufficiently severe symptoms, usually associated with local sepsis, haemorrhage or perforation, to justify admission. However, the variation in admission rates is so large that they should reflect true differences in overall frequency. Table 5.5 shows that a hundred-fold variation was detectable between Aberdeen in Scotland, and three tropical areas.[9] A greater

Table 5.5 Hospital admission rates per 100 000 population per year for diverticular disease in different areas.[9] (Abridged).

	Number of admissions	Admission rate
Aberdeen	206	12·8
Fiji: Fijian	1	0·21
Indian	2	0·34
Lagos	2	0·17
Singapore: Chinese	7	0·14
Malay	1	0·10

frequency of diverticulosis has been found in negro than in white populations in the same area, and in Mexico diverticula were not found in autopsies on the native Indian people, though they were detected in nearly one in ten of the Spanish population examined.[10]

Time trends It is frequently suggested that diverticular disease has become a common problem as this century has advanced. This opinion is based upon the demonstration that the mortality rate from diverticular disease has increased greatly in the last fifty years, and that diverticular disease has been detected clinically more often as time has passed.[11]

Crude death rates for diverticular disease have risen ten-fold in the last fifty years in England and Wales. However, this trend may be explained in part by the increasing proportion in the population of elderly individuals, who are more likely to have the condition. In addition, changing fashion in the pattern of certification of the cause of death could have increased the diverticular disease group. In the 1920s the increasing sophistication of radiological techniques was quickly followed by results showing that diverticula could be detected very frequently at barium enema. There is no way of knowing whether the rise in mortality rates and the increasing clinical demonstration of diverticula reflects a marked and continued rise in the real prevalence of the condition in white populations.

Predisposing factors

Diet The concept that a low dietary residue is the prime cause of diverticular disease through an association with a high intracolonic pressure has been strongly pressed. The epidemiological evidence in support derives from two sources, geographical comparisons and time trends. A constellation of complaints which includes appendicitis, piles, diverticulosis and large bowel cancer has been found to be common in white populations who, by and large, tend to take diets with a low unabsorbable residue.[11,12] In contrast, tropical African and other populations who take a relatively unrefined diet with a higher content of dietary fibre have a low frequency of all these complaints.

The time trend evidence is exemplified by the coincidence between the rise in mortality from diverticular disease and a postulated fall in dietary fibre content. Two main difficulties arise in accepting this evidence, firstly the data on ordinary dietary intakes from earlier periods is incomplete and secondly, the advent of the roller milling of flour in the 1880s which has been claimed to be a significant factor in reducing the fibre content of flour did not, in fact, seem to have such a marked effect as had been claimed (Table 5.6). Though the fibre content as cereal fibre fell there has been a

Table 5.6 Estimated dietary fibre content in different time periods in England.[26]

	Dietary fibre (g/day)	Percentage content as		
		Vegetables	Fruit and nuts	Cereals
1880	21·8	56	not known	44
1909–13	23·9	47	8	45
1942	32·0–37·5*	35	6	59
1957	23·3	50	13	37
1970	22·7	51	13	36

* Attributable to changes in dietary composition during the 1939–45 war.

simultaneous increase in fibre intake as vegetables, fruit and nuts. Whether this compensates biologically is unclear. Furthermore, when dietary fibre intake increased in the 1939 to 1945 war when wheat flour extraction procedures were altered, mortality rates from diverticular disease in England and Wales did not fall, though they had done six years earlier when flour extraction methods had not yet changed.[13,14]

These contradictory claims may partially arise through trying to make too much of inadequate evidence when the fibre content of the diet is poorly characterized. Crude fibre is a chemical entity which underestimates the total biological fibre content of the diet consisting of a series of complex polysaccharides.[15] On the other hand, total dietary fibre is hard to characterize, and the different varieties may well have heterogeneous effects.

The claim of an association between a low residue diet and liability to diverticular disease based upon comparative geographical findings looks more convincing. Though the data are limited in quantity, bowel transit times seem on average to be shorter, and stool weights to be greater in Africans living on traditional and semi-traditional diets than in Europeans taking refined diets (Table 5.7), and faecal bulk in European populations can, as might be

Table 5.7 Bowel transit time, daily faecal weight and dietary intake patterns.[6]

Subjects	Diet	Mean daily faecal weight in grams	Mean transit time in hours
South African, African rural schoolchildren	Unrefined	275	33·5
Uganda, rural villagers	Unrefined	470	35·7
South African, white students	Refined	173	48·0
United Kingdom, Naval ratings and wives	Refined	104	83·4

expected, be increased by adding non-absorbable carbohydrate. Further support for the fibre hypothesis would be derived if direct comparisons of dietary intakes in white populations showed that those who developed diverticulosis had had lower fibre intakes than those who did not. In general it seems likely that dietary fibre intake does affect liability to diverticular disease, and that such dietary deficiency is a prime causal factor, but the evidence could be strengthened.

Associated disease In countries where diverticular disease is common, large bowel cancer, appendicitis and haemorrhoids are also frequently found, and a basic underlying relationship with dietary fibre intake is claimed. Patients with diverticular disease are frequently claimed to be overweight, but this opinion is unsupported by factual evidence, though it is noteworthy that gallstones, which have been shown to be more prevalent in people who are overweight, do not seem to be especially common in those with diverticulosis.[4]

Appendicitis

Appendicectomy is the commonest emergency operation in Western Europe and in North America. The diagnosis of acute appendicitis is obvious when there is localized abdominal pain, fever and signs of peritoneal inflammation, for though the condition can still be mimicked by mesenteric lymphadenitis and acute ileitis in particular, the operative findings of an acutely inflamed and perhaps gangrenous appendix will confirm the clinical suspicion. However, there are lesser grades of inflammation which may be associated with recurrent pain reminiscent of appendicitis, so that an absolute distinction between the presence and absence of acute appendiceal inflammation is impossible. The same difficulties arise in histopathological examination, for cellular infiltration of the appendix is common, though its degree varies.

Death from appendicitis, particularly in the young, is a rarity, and the only satisfactory data on which to base epidemiological analyses of appendicitis are operative statistics, but then only when care has been taken to try and decide whether the organ is acutely diseased or not, there being a natural tendency to confirm the presence of appendicitis once the diagnosis has been made clinically.

Incidence: age, sex and social class distribution, and geographical frequency

Table 5.8 shows the admission rates recorded for appendicitis in England and Wales in 1973. The figures conform to the expected trend in that the disease has its greatest frequency between the ages

Table 5.8 Appendicitis: admission rates per 10 000 population in England and Wales, 1973.[16]

Age	Men	Women
0–4	3·5	3·0
5–14	39·0	32·5
15–19	41·3	50·9
20–24	29·2	33·0
25–34	18·5	20·1
35–44	10·9	11·6
45–64	7·4	7·8
65–74	6·1	5·6
75+	6·6	4·8

of 5 and 25 years, and equal proportions of men and women are affected.

This pattern probably characterizes that observed in Western Europe, in North America and Australasia, though data are fragmentary. By contrast, appendicitis is rare in tropical Africa, and in much of India. Though statistics in such countries are rudimentary the disease appears to be so rare that it is very unlikely that it is in fact common. Furthermore, in South Africa appendicitis in the Bantu appears to be a disease of those working in industrialized areas, and in Nigeria appendicitis again seems to be a disease of city dwellers. It has also been claimed that appendicitis became prevalent in African troops when they were given British Army rations.

In westernized populations appendicitis appears to be more common in the more affluent, thus when National Service recruits were examined in the 1950s appendicectomy has been performed in nearly twice as many who had had a grammar or independent school education as in those with the lower level of secondary modern education.[19] However, this difference could reflect differing social pressures over the need for investigation and treatment of abdominal pain, rather than a true difference in the frequency of appendicitis. Whether similar changes of social attitudes could explain the claimed increase in frequency of operations for appendicitis in negro communities and in migrants is more doubtful.

Predisposing factors

The dominant working hypothesis is that alterations in the non-absorbable residue in the diet influence liability to faecolith formation, and hence to acute appendicitis.

The evidence in favour of this hypothesis derives in part from pathophysiological considerations and in part from epidemiological features of the disease. The pathophysiological changes include the frequency with which faecoliths can be demonstrated in acute appendicitis, and the characteristically distal distribution in the appendix of any inflammatory changes suggesting an association with faecal stasis.

The epidemiological evidence is based upon geographical and time trend analyses of appendix frequency.

Time trends Burkitt has argued persuasively that an increase in the frequency of appendicitis has taken place in the last hundred years, and that this can be associated with the adoption of a low residue diet.[18] This suggestion is not new, having been put forward in 1920 by Rendle Short.[20] Appendicitis was an unrecognized condition until 1886, when Fitz described its characteristic features as an acute illness.[17] Hitherto an ill-defined entity of perityphlitis was accepted, but in the closing years of the nineteenth century acute appendicitis was accepted as an illness. There was then a rapid rise from an occasionally described condition to a common illness and it seems likely that this increase represented a real increase in disease frequency rather than a change of classification.

Accurate statistics of the frequency of true acute appendicitis, as opposed to the frequency of appendicectomy, are unlikely to be obtainable because it is impossible to decide what proportion of patients operated upon did indeed have acute inflammatory changes in the appendix.

Recently it has been suggested that the frequency of acute appendicitis has fallen in the USA, and hospital discharges and deaths ascribed to the disease have also fallen in the United Kingdom, as has the frequency of sickness absence from work.[21-23] However, the fall in frequency in England and Wales has been accompanied by a rise in admissions with abdominal pain of uncertain cause, suggesting that reclassification may be at least as important as changes in the frequency of appendicitis (Fig. 5.1).

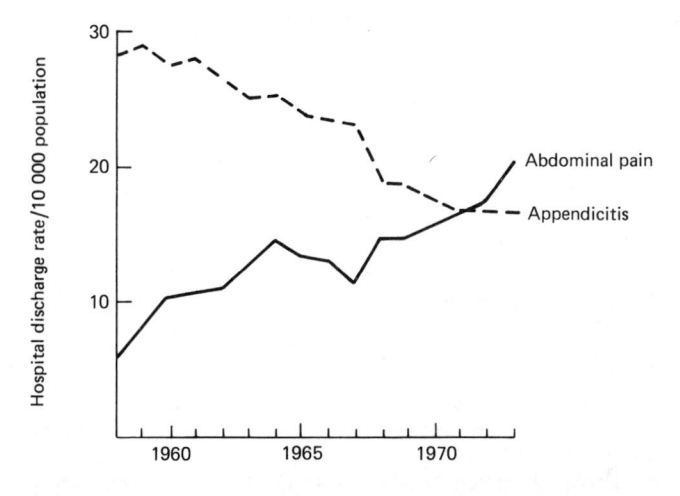

Fig. 5.1 The changing admission rate for appendicitis and abdominal pain of uncertain cause in England and Wales 1958–73

Diet Coincident with the claimed increase in frequency of appendicitis in the last hundred years, it has been suggested that there was a fall in the dietary content of unabsorbable residue. Proponents of this view have proposed that increasing affluence and industrialization were associated with these changes, which were due, for instance, in part to the advent of roller milling of flour. The hypothesis may be correct, but supportive evidence is hard to obtain. Robertson[13] has suggested that there may have been no change in dietary fibre content in the United Kingdom in the last hundred years, as measured by crude fibre intake. In addition an analysis of dietary fibre intake by questionnaire in control patients and in those with appendicitis failed to show any differences as measured by crude fibre intake, though the proportions of fruit, cereals and nuts did vary to some extent.[24] However, the chemically defined entity of crude fibre may bear little relationship to the biologically available fibre. More recently it has been suggested that though the total fibre intake in the diet may have changed little in the last hundred years, the proportion derived from cereals may have fallen. If this is so then the change seems to be modest,[26] and its significance is unclear.

A tendency for appendicitis to be common in the more affluent in England has been ascribed to the refined diets of the better-off, and in Switzerland, a fall in the frequency of appendicitis during the Second World War has been ascribed to the widespread adoption of vegetarian diets.[25]

There is a clear need to obtain better epidemiological information about the characteristics of people who develop acute appendicitis, and about the features of their antecedent diets.

References

1. Mendeloff, A. I., Dunn, J. P. (1971). *Digestive Diseases.* Cambridge Mass., Harvard University Press.
2. Dearlove, T. P. (1954). Diverticulitis and diverticulosis, with a report on a rare complication. *Medical Journal of Australia* **1,** 470–5.
3. Manoussos, O. N., Truelove, S. C., Lumsden, K. (1967). Prevalence of colonic diverticulosis in the general population of Oxford area. *British Medical Journal* **3,** 762–3.
4. Hughes, L. E. (1969). Post-mortem survey of diverticular disease of the colon. *Gut* **10,** 336–51.
5. Eastwood, M. A., Sanderson, Jean, Pocock, S. J., Mitchell, W. D. (1977). Variation of the incidence of diverticular disease with the City of Edinburgh. *Gut* **18,** 571–4.
6. Painter, N. S. (1975). *Diverticular Disease of the Colon – a Deficiency Disease of Western Civilization.* London, Heinemann.
7. Köhler, R. (1968). The incidence of colonic diverticulosis in Finland and Sweden. *Acta chirurgica Scandinavica* **126,** 148–55.
8. Havia, T. (1971). Diverticulosis of the colon. *Acta chirurgica Scandinavica* **137,** 367–73.
9. Kyle, J., Adesola, A. O., Tinckler, L. F., De Beaux, J. (1967). Incidence of diverticulitis. *Scandinavian Journal of Gastroenterology* **2,** 77–80.
10. De la Vega, J. M. (1976). Diverticular disease of the colon. In *Gastroenterology,* Vol. II, ed. Bockus, H. L. Philadelphia, Saunders.
11. Painter, N. S., Burkitt, D. P. (1975). Diverticular disease of the colon, a 20th Century problem. *Clinics in Gastroenterology* **4,** 3–21.
12. Burkitt, D. P., Walker, A. R. P., Painter, N. S. (1972). Effect of dietary fibre on stools and transit times, and its role in the causation of disease. *Lancet* **2,** 1408–12.
13. Robertson, J. (1972). Change in the fibre content of the British diet. *Nature* **238,** 290–1.
14. Eastwood, M. A., Fisher, N., Greenwood, C. T., Hutchinson, J. B. (1974). Perspectives on the bran hypothesis. *Lancet* **1,** 1029–33.

15. Cummings, J. (1973). Dietary fibre. *Gut* **14**, 69–81.
16. *Report on the Hospital In-Patient Enquiry for the year 1973* (1977). London, HMSO.
17. Fitz, R. H. (1886). Perforating inflammation of the vermiform appendix: with special reference to early diagnosis and treatment. *American Journal of Medical Science* **92**, 321–66.
18. Burkitt, D. P. (1971). The aetiology of appendicitis. *British Journal of Surgery* **58**, 695–9.
19. Lee, J. A. H. (1957). An association between social circumstances and appendicitis in young people. *British Medical Journal* **1**, 1217–19.
20. Short, A. R. (1920). The causation of appendicitis. *British Journal of Surgery* **8**, 171–88.
21. Castleton, K. B., Puestow, C. B., Sauer, D. (1959). Is appendicitis decreasing in frequency? *Archives of Surgery* **78**, 794–8.
22. Taylor, P. (1974). Sickness absence: facts and misconceptions. *Journal of the Royal College of Physicians of London* **8**, 315–33.
23. Howie, J. G. R. (1966). Deaths from appendicitis and appendicectomy. *Lancet* **2**, 1334–7.
24. Cove-Smith, J. R., Langman, M. J. S. (1975). Appendicitis and dietary fibre. *Gut* **16**, 409.
25. Fleisch, A. (1946). Nutrition in Switzerland during the war. *Schweizerische Medizinische Wochenschrift* **76**, 889–93.
26. Southgate, D. A. T., Bingham, J., Robertson, J. (1978). Dietary fibre in the British diet. *Nature* **274**, 51–2.

6
Gallstones

Gallstones contain varying proportions of cholesterol and bile pigments together with a number of other substances including calcium and magnesium salts, bile acids and other organic compounds. It has been conventional to distinguish between pigment and cholesterol stones clinically, but this separation is in part artificial. Pigment stones contain relatively more pigment, but also appreciable and often large amounts of cholesterol; whilst cholesterol stones likewise can contain appreciably large amounts of bile pigments.[1] Nevertheless the attempt to distinguish broad groups of primarily cholesterol stones and primarily pigment stones is useful because aetiological factors are likely to differ. In practice few epidemiological studies have distinguished between the different clinical varieties of stone. No information is available about the presence or absence of cholecystitis in association with the stones, although stones can develop in the absence of gall bladder inflammation, and the role of biliary infection in causing gallstones is still poorly understood.

Epidemiological analyses are also hampered by the difficulties of deciding exactly how frequent gallstones are. Symptomatic gallstones are probably outnumbered by asymptomatic gallstones, and therefore reliance upon operative or clinical diagnostic criteria must underestimate true frequency rates. Few people die with gallstone disease, and death rates, as with peptic ulcer, could reflect the quality of medical care rather than the problem of the underlying condition. Reliance therefore has to be placed upon necropsy data, (which, especially in the young, cannot be assumed to be derived from a random population sample),[3,4] from a limited number of cholecystographic surveys,[2,5] and from a judicious examination of clinical and mortality data.

The pathophysiological changes which induce gallstones to develop are poorly understood. Patients with cholesterol stones tend to have bile which is supersaturated with cholesterol, but the precise reasons why stones should develop at any one time are unclear. Though pigment stones contain relatively high proportions of bile pigments, the bile itself does not contain unusually large amounts of pigment, and, for instance in those with haemolytic anaemia, the proportions of unconjugated bilirubin entering the bile may still be very low.

Age and sex distribution

Gallstones are in general more common in women than men, and Table 6.1 shows this trend in autopsy surveys in Scandinavia and

Table 6.1 Autopsy frequency of gallstones.[3,4]

Age	Percentage with stones		
	Oslo	Malmo	Prague
Men			
30–39	2	5	7
40–49	3	15	15
50–59	9	21	17
60–69	13	28	31
70–79	16	34	40
80–89	22	42	35
90+	31	61	54
Women			
30–39	3	28	27
40–49	8	24	15
50–59	17	39	36
60–69	24	53	51
70–79	35	61	55
80–89	38	60	59
90+	34	57	60

Czechoslovakia.[3,4] In addition in these areas the difference in sex incidence disappeared as patients became older. The findings can be contrasted with the experience in Framingham, Massachusetts,[5] where new cases of gallstones were consistently more frequent in

Table 6.2 Gallbladder disease in Framingham, Massachusetts.[5]

Age	10 year incidence rate per 1000			10 year prevalence rate per 1000		
	Men	Women	Ratio	Men	Women	Ratio
30–39	11	30	1:2·7	12	52	1:4·3
40–49	30	66	1:2·2	39	123	1:3·2
50–62	48	89	1:1·9	79	181	1:2·3

Gallstones

women than men, whatever their age (Table 6.2), though the disparity in sex ratio tended to diminish as time passed. There is no means of knowing whether the variations recorded between these surveys are due to differing methods of data collection, the European results being obtained at autopsy and the US data as presentations of gall bladder disease, or whether they reflect true differences, perhaps in association with obesity or parity. Cholelithiasis may also be more likely to be symptomless in the elderly, so that the US data could tend generally to underestimate stone frequency.

Clinical experience suggests that gallstone frequency increases in women with parity, and this trend is borne out by epidemiological data as well as by clinical surveys. Horn[6] and van der Linden[7] found more married than single women to have gallstones, and in general, particularly in younger women, stones tended to occur in those who had borne children. There have been similar findings in the USA (Table 6.3), but no clear relationship could be established with the

Table 6.3 Pregnancy and liability to gallstones (abridged).[5]

Previous pregnancies	Number with gallstones	
	Observed	Expected
Nil	32	38·5
1–2	48	54·3
3–4	50	44·2
5 or more	28	22·2

numbers of children born. In Pima Indians who have much gallstone disease there is an association with parity, though this is insufficient in itself to explain the occurrence of stones.[16,17]

Time trends

It is generally believed that gallstones have increased in frequency in Europe and North America with time. Difficulties arise in examining such data because it is hard to be sure that the trends found do not reflect increasing diagnostic awareness. Increases in frequency are recorded in Scandinavia, in England, in North America and in Japan. Examination of the frequency of operations for gall bladder disease in Bristol, England,[8] over a forty-year period showed a quadrupling of frequency (Table 6.4). This was not explained by a tendency for less severe gallstone disease to be operated upon as time passed or by increasing age in the general population, and the authors concluded that a true rise in frequency of gallstones was likely. Comparison of the frequency of gall bladder

Table 6.4 Operations for gallstones in Bristol, England.[8]

Age	Percentage distribution		
	1933	1950	1970
Up to 29	3·6	4·0	9·3
30–59	64·5	56·9	52·3
60+	31·9	39·1	38·4
Total number	153	231	623

operations in Luton, England, Windsor, Ontario and Rennes, France[9] has shown a doubling of the frequency of cholecystectomy over a time span as short as ten years. An anomalous and unexplained finding was a tendency of patients in Canada to be relatively thin. In Japan a falling frequency of pigment stones has been matched by a rising frequency of cholesterol stones in those living in urban areas which has been attributed to the adoption of a western life-style.[10,11] Whether gallstones have increased in frequency in western countries is still questioned, either on the grounds that differences in operation frequency simply reflect differing attitudes to the need for operation,[12] or because no evidence of an increased frequency has been found.[13]

Geographical incidence and ethnic variation

The generally accepted pattern of gallstone prevalence is of a high frequency in Northern Europe and North America amongst white populations, with lower frequencies in most tropical areas, such as tropical Africa.[14,15] In many areas the overall prevalence of gallstones is inadequately described, and this may be because stones are rare (as is probably the case in Central Africa), because medical services are poorly developed, or because the special attention which is needed to get reliable estimates of stone prevalence has never been given to the condition.

Comparative estimates of stone prevalence within different areas of Northern Europe and North America are hard to make because survey techniques may differ. Basically similar prevalence rates were recorded in Sweden and Czechoslovakia by autopsy studies (Table 6.1), whereas rates in Norway were half those in Sweden. This difference may be real but the assumption that autopsy findings reflect the true population frequency of gallstones is not necessarily justified.

The frequency of cholecystectomy in Windsor, Ontario was six times higher than in Luton, England, or Rennes, France, and nine times higher in women under the age of 35.[9] The reasons for this difference are unclear. There is no means of knowing whether it reflects a generally greater prevalence of stones in North America than in Northern Europe, or a differing attitude to investigation and the need for cholecystectomy.

Within North American populations there are fluctuations in gallstone frequency in different racial groups. The Pima Indians are considerably more liable to gallstones than other populations,[16,17] and in women it is the exception for an individual to be gallstone-free (Table 6.5). Again, the reasons are unclear; the stones are of

Table 6.5 Gallstones in Pima Indians.[16]

Age	Percentage with gallstones by cholecystography	
	Men	Women
15–24	0	13
25–34	4	73
35–44	11	71
45–54	32	76
55–64	66	62
65+	68	90

cholesterol type, and bile tends to be supersaturated with cholesterol. Correction of stone incidence for parity does not reduce the frequency to that observed in white populations.

By contrast, a consistently lower gallstone frequency has been found in black Americans than in white Americans, in Bantu living in Johannesburg than in white South Africans, and in black Panamanians than in white residents (Table 6.6).[18–21] The differ-

Table 6.6 Incidence of gallstones in white and coloured populations.

	Percentage with gallstones at autopsy			
	Men		Women	
	White	Black	White	Black
USA[18,19]	10	3	22	9
	7	2	11	5
Panama[20]	17	8	9	5
South Africa[21]	10	1	20	4

ences are probably due in part to a tendency for gallstone disease to be more prevalent in those of higher socio-economic status. This view is mainly based upon standardized mortality ratios which have been consistently high in men of higher economic status in the USA

Table 6.7 Standardized mortality ratios for gallstone disease in the USA[22] and the UK.[23]

	Social class				
	I	II	III	IV	V
UK					
Men aged 15–64					
1949–53	243	136	89	73	82
1959–63	123	96	108	89	93
Married women					
1949–53	97	87	93	117	126
1959–63	56	71	105	111	147
USA					
White men aged 20–64	–	130	110	93	79

(*N.B.*: Occupational classification is not completely identical in the two countries.)

and in the United Kingdom (Table 6.7), though somewhat confusingly the opposite trend has been detected in wives according to social class.[22,23] That mortality data can parallel incidence rates is suggested by the high mortality rates for gallstones in the mountain states of the USA, where there is a substantial Indian population.[24] The distribution of gallstones in other non-white populations is poorly understood. In India itself they are probably commoner in the North than the South, the pattern being the converse of that for duodenal ulcer.[25] In Thailand gallstones have been recorded twice as commonly in the Chinese as in the remaining population.[26] Gallstones in Japan now seem to be of two types, mainly pigmented stones in rural areas and predominantly cholesterol stones in cities where previously most were pigment stones. During chemical analyses of gallstones from different countries Sutor and Wooley found those from Germany, Austria and Sweden to be similar, whereas there was a tendency for calcium carbonate stones (a minor proportion of the total) to be more common in England. In India there was an increase in the proportion of calcium phosphate and in South Africa more calcium phosphate and palmitate but less cholesterol.[27,28]

Comparative analyses of bile composition are similarly fragmentary. In white Western populations, bile tends to be saturated or supersaturated with cholesterol.[29] A direct comparison between bile samples obtained in Japan and the USA suggested that in the USA cholesterol phospholipid and bilirubin concentrations were increased in the bile despite the greater frequency of pigment stones in Japan.[11] The Pima Indians of the USA have been found to have a reduced bile acid pool, a fast turnover of bile acids and inadequate synthetic rates with possibly a defect of reabsorption, the reasons being unclear.[30,31] The findings in Pima Indians can be contrasted with those in the Masai of East Africa, who derive two-thirds of their calorie intake from fat, but rarely develop gallstones and have bile undersaturated for cholesterol.

Information about the frequency of gallstones in migrants is sketchy. Japanese who move to Hawaii are probably more prone to cholesterol stones than those who continue to live in Japan,[32] and the frequency of gallstones in the urban Bantu of South Africa, though lower than in urban whites, is probably much higher than in the rural Bantu population.[14,15,21]

Diet

It is generally assumed that dietary changes are of prime importance in influencing the frequency of gallstones. Though this may seem self-evident, the supporting evidence is weak.

The tendency for gallstones, and particularly cholesterol stones, to occur in people who are overweight, and in people who live in Western Europe and the USA, suggests an association with increased food consumption.

Case-control studies have given divergent results. In Australia, patients with gallstones and control individuals seemed to have equal caloric intakes though the gallstone patients ate less fat, a difference which suggests that the dietary questionnaires elicited information about current habits rather than about customs at a time when gallstones were developing.[33] By contrast, in France, the same technique suggested that stones tended to develop in people with an increased caloric intake irrespective of dietary composition, a result which might have been predicted from knowledge that gallstone patients tend to be overweight.[34] The same French group also found a tendency for biliary cholesterol concentrations to be correlated with dietary caloric intake.[35] In the USA, as in Australia, no correlation was detected between dietary fat, protein or carbohydrate intake in gallstone patients compared with controls, though there was a slight negative correlation with alcohol intake.[5]

Somewhat confusingly, post-mortem studies have suggested that gallstones may be common in individuals taking blood cholesterol-lowering diets as a preventive measure in ischaemic heart disease compared with control individuals on ordinary diets containing similar proportions of fat.[36]

Geographical comparisons are few; a rising incidence of cholesterol stone disease in urban Japanese has been attributed to the adoption of Western dietary patterns, whilst in India a high incidence of gallstones in railway workers in the North has been correlated with a diet which contains large amounts of saturated fats. This high frequency has been contrasted with a lower figure in South India where total fat intake is low.[25] However, such a pattern does not seem to obtain generally, because the Masai of East Africa rarely develop gallstones despite a diet rich in animal fat.[37] Finally, Pima Indian communities in the United States have an extremely high incidence of gallstones and tend to be overweight, but the incidence of gallstones in them does not correlate directly with the degree to which they are overweight, although biliary cholesterol secretion rates seem to correlate with the degree to which they are overweight.[17]

The main consistent feature seems to be the association between obesity and gallstones, together with a generally high frequency of gallstones in Western Europe and North America. In addition there is a suggestion of an inverse correlation between factors causing pigment and cholesterol stone disease. The underlying reasons are unclear. Heaton has emphasized that diets rich in refined carbohydrates such as sucrose can be used experimentally to induce gallstones and considers that a high energy intake associated with such diets, which are widely taken in Europe and North America, induces hepatic cholesterol synthesis and secretion into the bile.[38] Direct evidence to support this hypothesis is lacking and the use of deliberate dietary intervention policies, such as those recommended in the management of ischaemic heart disease, as means of examining the factors causing gallstones has been insufficiently exploited.

Predisposing diseases

Though gallstones are common, there are few well proven associations between their development and the presence of other diseases.

Cirrhosis An increased frequency of gallstones has been detected in patients with hepatic cirrhosis.[39] Post-mortem analyses suggest that there is approximately a doubling of frequency compared with the frequency overall in patients dying with other diseases. Stones tend to be of the pigment type and in one survey an equal frequency was found in men and women, with no increase in incidence with advancing age. The mechanism is unclear: total bilirubin output seems if anything to be decreased, so that some more sophisticated explanation than a direct quantitative relationship is needed.

Degenerative vascular disease The tendency of gallstone patients to be overweight has suggested that stones should be more frequent in those with raised serum cholesterol concentrations, in those with hyperlipoproteinaemia and in those with atherosclerosis. There is little evidence to support such associations. Epidemiological studies[5,17,58] have failed to show that individuals with gallstones tend to have high serum cholesterol concentrations, nor that those who have high serum cholesterol concentrations are unduly liable to later gallstone development (Table 6.8). However, in one study of

Table 6.8 Gallstones and serum cholesterol concentrations in men aged 30–62 years.[5]

	Number	Mean serum cholesterol concentration (mg %)
Patients developing gallstones	66	225·1
Patients not developing gallstones	2173	223·9

hyperlipoproteinaemic patients, more gallstones have been detected in those with type IV hyperlipoproteinaemia (hyperprebeta) than in those with type II. The frequencies of gallstones were 41% in men and 68% in women with type IV, compared with 13% in men and 22% in women with type II.[40] In addition, a tendency towards higher serum triglyceride (and cholesterol) concentrations was noted in one study in gallstone patients compared with matched controls, though the numbers studied were small.[59]

No clear association with degenerative vascular disease has been detected. One autopsy investigation suggested a correlation between the occurrence of gallstones and the presence of cerebrovascular disease in elderly men and women, and between gallstones and coronary heart disease in elderly women, but no association was found with aortic atherosclerosis, and where trends were detectable they were slight.[41] Other analyses have failed to reveal any trends at all.

Diabetes mellitus Despite earlier claims to the contrary, surveys of gallstone frequency have in general failed to show any association with hyperglycaemia, and negative results have been found in the United States[5] and in the autopsy studies in Prague and Malmö.[3]

Haemolytic disease General clinical evidence supports the existence of associations between haemolytic diseases such as spherocytosis, sickle cell anaemia and haemolysis after heart valve replacement and liability to pigment stones.[1,42] However, even when all such conditions are taken into consideration they still only account for a minority of all pigment stones detected. The mechanism of stone formation is unclear: most bilirubin is secreted as soluble conjugates and examination of pigment stone biles has shown no increase in bile pigment concentrations compared with normal biles, though the small proportion of unconjugated bilirubin usually detectable in bile may be increased.

Hyperparathyroidism An association has been claimed in the past between hyperparathyroidism and gallstone disease. The suggestion has probably been due to an inadequate understanding of the general frequency of gallstones. When this is taken into account, no increase in gallstone frequency is detectable.[43-45]

Hyperlipoproteinaemia Despite the indifferent evidence in favour of an association between gallstones and atherosclerosis, in one study gallstones were found three times as often in patients with type IV hyperlipoproteinaemia (hyperprebeta) as in type IIa.[40] The significance of this finding is unclear.

Infections of the biliary tree Strictures and other conditions predisposing to bile stasis are commonly supposed to predispose to pigment stones. Convincing evidence to support such an association is hard to obtain, but stones have been found commonly in the intrahepatic ducts of patients with lower ductal strictures.

Biliary infection with *Escherichia coli*, and the presence of ascariasis, have been suggested as causes of pigment stones in Japan. The mechanism proposed is deglucuronidation of bilirubin conjugates by bacterial glucuronidase giving an insoluble nidus for stone formation.[46] This hypothesis is supported by the finding that pigment stone biles in Japan are usually infected with *E. coli*, which produces β-glucuronidase, and calcium bilirubinate can be precipitated from bile by the addition of this enzyme. However, in the United States and Western Europe, though pigment stones form about a quarter of all stones, the bile is usually sterile so that the bacterial degradation hypothesis may not be universally applicable. Alternative sources of glucuronidase are the liver or gall bladder themselves, but proof that such enzyme activity accounts for the development of pigment stones in western countries is lacking, and other candidates exist. These include increased sulphated glycoprotein output, possibly giving sites for pigment stone precipitation, and at least in some patients, increased unconjugated bilirubin concentrations.[1] Pigment stone formation in the USA has been found to be associated with high biliary concentrations of unconjugated bilirubin presumably due to direct secretion into bile since bacterial infection was undetectable.[60]

Ileal disease and resection A high proportion of patients with ileal disease or resection have been found to have gallstones. In an initial study in Bristol, Heaton and Read[47] detected gallstones in nearly one-third of all patients with these conditions, but the proportions rose to three-quarters if only those with ileal disease or resections of at least fifteen years' duration were considered. Confirmatory evidence of an increase has been obtained elsewhere in the United Kingdom in Leeds, where gallstones were found three times as

124 *Gallstones*

commonly as expected, and in the USA.[48-49] The likely mechanism is an interruption of normal ileal reabsorption of bile salts with a consequential fall in bile salt concentrations in the bile because compensatory hepatic synthesis is inadequate.

Obesity Individuals who are overweight have an increased liability to gallstones, and Table 6.9, drawn from the data of the

Table 6.9 Body weight and gallstone frequency.[5]

Relative weight	Number with gallstones			
	Men		Women	
	Observed	Expected	Observed	Expected
<90	7	12·6	28	33·1
90–109	39	35·4	68	74·8
110+	20	17·4	64	51·1

Framingham survey[5] illustrates this point. The reasons for the association are unclear, but it has been suggested that fat people tend to have high biliary cholesterol concentrations. An association of gallstones with obesity may in part explain the tendency for gallstone mortality to be greater in those of high socio-economic status.

Pancreatitis Pancreatitis commonly develops in people with gallstones, and the clinical suggestion is that gallstones predispose to pancreatitis. No evidence exists to support the reverse hypothesis.

Drug-induced gallstones Little information is available to suggest that drug intake influences the occurrence of gallstones, but this simply reflects the paucity of searches made.

Examination of the frequency of gallstone disease in women taking sex hormones, either as oestrogens post-menopausally or as oral contraceptives, has revealed an increased frequency of gallstones: the change is of the order of a doubling. It is presumably attributable to changes in bile composition, thus cholesterol saturation of bile is increased in those taking oral contraceptives.[52,53,55] In Sweden, in Falun and Gothenberg, cholecystectomy was performed more often in 1971 than in 1961, there being 606 such operations in 1961 and 1003 in 1971.[54] The increase in operations was greater in women than in men, and was particularly prominent in those of child-bearing age which has been taken to suggest a relationship with the use of oral contraceptives, though no direct evidence was obtained to support the contention. The claim of a particular increase in frequency of gallstones in younger women is at variance with earlier results from the country suggesting that any increase was especially marked in men, though these data substantially antedated the period when oral contraceptives were freely used.

Small increases in gallstone frequency have been noted in patients taking drugs intended to lower serum cholesterol concentrations, including clofibrate and oestrogens,[50,51] clofibrate being thought to raise biliary cholesterol levels. Lesser changes of doubtful significance in individuals taking nicotinic acid and dextrothroxine were also noted.

Hereditary factors

The widely held clinical impression that hereditary factors influence the occurrence of gallstones is poorly supported. Several investigations have shown a high frequency of gallstones amongst the relatives of gallstone patients, but these may be no more than chance findings. However, a higher frequency of gallstones has been found in the families of affected patients than in control families, and a trend towards greater concordance in monozygotic than in dizygotic twins has been detected.[56] No individual genetic marker has been found to be associated with gallstones, and, in particular, the ABO blood groups have shown no consistent variation in pattern in those with gallstones.[57]

References

1. Soloway, R. D., Trotman, B. W., Ostrow, J. D. (1977). Pigment gallstones. *Gastroenterology* **72,** 167–82.
2. Bainton, D., Davies, G. T., Evans, K. T., Gravelle, I. H. (1976). Gall bladder disease prevalence in a South Wales industrial town. *New England Journal of Medicine* **294,** 1147–69.
3. Zahar, Z., Sternby, H. M., Kagan, A., Uemura, K., Vanecek, R., Vichert, A. M. (1974). Frequency of cholelithiasis in Prague and Malmö. An autopsy study. *Scandinavian Journal of Gastroenterology* **9,** 3–7.
4. Torvik, A., Høivik, B. (1960). Gallstones in an autopsy series: incidence, complications, and correlations with carcinoma of the gall bladder. *Acta Chirurgica Scandinavica* **120,** 168–74.
5. Friedman, G. D., Kannel, W. B., Dawber, K. R. (1966). The epidemiology of gall bladder disease: observations in the Framingham study. *Journal of Chronic Diseases* **19,** 273–92.
6. Horn, G. (1956). Observations in the aetiology of cholelithiasis. *British Medical Journal* **2,** 732–7.
7. Van der Linden, W. (1961). Some biological traits in female gallstone-disease patients. *Acta Chirurgica Scandinavica,* suppl. 269, 1–94.
8. Holland, C., Heaton, K. W. (1972). Increasing frequency of gall bladder operations in the Bristol clinical area. *British Medical Journal* **3,** 672–5.

9. Plant, J. C. D., Percy, I., Bates, T., Gastard, J., de Nercy, H. Y. (1973). Incidence of gall bladder disease in Canada, England and France. Lancet 2, 249–51.
10. Nakayama, F., Miyake, H. (1970). Changing state of gallstone disease in Japan. Composition of the stones and treatment of the condition. American Journal of Surgery 120, 794.
11. Nakayama, F., van der Linden, W. (1970). Bile composition: Sweden versus Japan. American Journal of Surgery 122, 8–12.
12. Opit, L. J., Greenhill, S. (1974). Prevalence of gallstones in relation to differing treatment rates for biliary disease. British Journal of Preventive and Social Medicine 28, 268–72.
13. Bateson, M. C., Bouchier, I. A. D. (1975). Prevalence of gallstones in Dundee; a necropsy study. British Medical Journal 4, 427–30.
14. Owor, R. (1964). Gallstones in the autopsy population at Mulago Hospital, Kampala. East African Medical Journal 41, 251–3.
15. Shaper, A. G., Patel, K. M. (1964). Diseases of the biliary tract in Africans in Uganda. East African Medical Journal 41, 251–3.
16. Sampliner, R. E., Bennett, P. H., Comess, L. J., Rose, F. A., Burch, T. A. (1970). Gall bladder disease in Pima Indians: demonstration of high prevalence and early onset by cholecystography. New England Journal of Medicine 283, 1358–64.
17. Comess, L. J., Bennett, P. J., Burch, T. A. (1967). Clinical gall bladder disease in the Pima Indians. New England Journal of Medicine 277, 894–8.
18. Lieber, M. M. (1952). The incidence of gallstones and their correlation with other diseases. Annals of Surgery 135, 394–405.
19. Cunningham, J. A., Hardenbergh, F. E. (1956). Comparative incidence of cholelithiasis in the Negro and White races. Archives of Internal Medicine 97, 68–72.
20. Hall, R. (1963). Incidence of gallstones in residents of the Panama Canal Zone. Surgery 53, 621–4.
21. Becker, B. J. P., Chatgidakis, C. B. (1952). Carcinoma of the gall bladder and cholelithiasis on the Witwatersrand. An autopsy survey of the racial incidence. South African Journal of Medical Science 3, 13–22.
22. Guralnick, L. (1963). Mortality by occupational level and cause of death among men 20 to 64 years of age: United States, 1950. Vital Statistics. Special Reports 53, 439.
23. Registrar General's Decennial Supplements: Occupational Mortality Tables for 1949–53, 1959–63. (1958, 1971). London, HMSO.
24. Mendeloff, A. I., Dunn, J. P. (1971). Digestive Diseases. Vital and Health Statistics Monographs. American Public Health Association. Cambridge, Mass., Harvard University Press.
25. Malhotra, S. L. (1968). Epidemiological study of cholelithiasis among railroad workers in India with special reference to causation. Gut 9, 290–5.
26. Stitnimankarn, T. (1960). The necropsy incidence of gallstones in Thailand. American Journal of the Medical Sciences 240, 349–52.
27. Sutor, D. J., Wooley, S. E. (1971). A statistical survey of the composition of gallstones in eight countries. Gut 12, 55–64.
28. Sutor, D. J., Wooley, S. E. (1973). The nature and incidence of gallstones containing calcium. Gut 14, 215–20.

29. Redinger, P. N., Small, D. M. (1972). Bile composition, bile salt metabolism and gallstones. *Archives of Internal Medicine* **130**, 618–30.
30. Grundy, S. M., Metzger, A. L., Adler, R. D. (1972). Mechanisms of lithogenic bile formation in American Indian women with cholesterol gallstones. *Journal of Clinical Investigation* **51**, 3026–43.
31. Vlahcevic, Z. R., Bell, C. C. Jr., Gregory, D. H., Buker, G., Juttijudata, P., Swell, L. (1972). Relationship of bile acid pool size to the formation of lithogenic bile in female Indians of the South-West. *Gastroenterology* **62**, 73–83.
32. Yamase, H., McNamara, J. J. (1972). Geographic differences in the incidence of gall bladder disease. Influence of environment and ethnic background. *American Journal of Surgery* **123**, 667–70.
33. Wheeler, M., Hill, L. L., Laby, B. (1970). Cholelithiasis: a clinical and dietary survey. *Gut* **11**, 430–7.
34. Sarles, H., Chabert, C., Pommeau, Y., Save, E., Mouret, H., Gérolami, A. (1969). Diet and cholesterol gallstones. *American Journal of Digestive Diseases* **14**, 531–7.
35. Sarles, H., Hauton, J. C., Lafont, H., Teissier, N., Planchier, N. E., Gérolami, A. (1968). Role de l'alimentation sur la concentration du cholestérol biliare chez l'homme lithiasique et non-lithiasique. *Clinica Chimica Acta* **19**, 147–55.
36. Sturdevant, R. A. L., Pearce, M. L., Dayton, S. (1973). Increased prevalence of cholelithiasis in men ingesting a serum-cholesterol-lowering diet. *New England Journal of Medicine* **288**, 24–7.
37. Biss, K., Ho, K-J., Mikkelson, B., Lewis, L., Taylor, C. B. (1971). Some unique biologic characteristics of the Masai of East Africa. *New England Journal of Medicine* **284**, 694–9.
38. Heaton, K. W. (1975). Gall stones and cholecystitis. In *Refined carbohydrate foods and disease*, ed. Burkitt, D. P. and Trowell, H. C. London, Academic Press.
39. Bouchier, I. A. D. (1969). Post-mortem study of the frequency of gallstones in patients with cirrhosis of the liver. *Gut* **10**, 705–10.
40. Einarrson, K., Hellstrom, K., Kallner, M. (1975). Gall bladder disease in hyperlipoproteinaemia. *Lancet* **1**, 484–7.
41. Sternby, N. H. (1968). Atherosclerosis in a defined population: an autopsy study in Malmö, Sweden. *Acta Pathologica et Microbiologica Scandinavica*. suppl. 194, 136–42.
42. Merendino, K. A., Manhas, D. R. (1973). Man-made gallstones: a new entity following cardiac valve replacement. *Annals of Surgery* **177**, 694–703.
43. Christensson, T., Einarrson, K. (1977). Cholelithiasis in subjects with hypercalcaemia and primary hyperparathyroidism. *Gut* **18**, 543–6.
44. Funk, C., Ammann, R., Binswanger, U., Mayor, G., Bihrer, R., Clavadetscher, P., Fumagalli, I., Leeman, A., Seiler, P., Stuby, K. (1974). Cholelithiasis beim primären Hyperparathyreoidismus. *Schweizerische Medizinische Wochenschrift* **104**, 1060–4.
45. Selle, J. G., Altemeier, W. A., Fullen, W. D., Goldsmith, R. E. (1972). Cholelithiasis in hyperparathyroidism. A neglected manifestation. *Archives of Surgery* **105**, 369–74.
46. Maki, T. (1961). Cholelithiasis in the Japanese. *Archives of Surgery* **82**, 599–612.

47. Heaton, K. W., Read, A. E. (1969). Gallstones in patients with disorders of the terminal ileum and disturbed bile salt metabolism. *British Medical Journal* **3,** 494–6.
48. Cohen, S., Kaplan, M., Gottlieb, C., Patterson, J. (1971). Liver disease and gallstones in regional enteritis. *Gastroenterology* **60,** 237–45.
49. Hill, G. L., Mair, W. S. J., Goligher, J. C. (1975). Gallstones after ileostomy and ileal resection. *Gut* **16,** 932–6.
50. Cooper, J., Geizerova, H., Oliver, M. F. (1975). Clofibrate and gallstones. *Lancet* **1,** 1083.
51. Gordon, R. S., Forman, S., Canner, P., Berge, K., Miller, D. (1977). Gall bladder disease as a wide effect of drugs influencing lipid metabolism. *New England Journal of Medicine* **296,** 1185–90.
52. Bennion, L. J., Ginsberg, R. L., Garnick, N. B., Bennett, P. H. (1976). Effects of oral contraceptives on the gall bladder bile of normal women. *New England Journal of Medicine* **294,** 189–92.
53. Boston Collaborative Drug Surveillance Program (1974). Surgically confirmed gall bladder disease, venous thromboembolism, and breast tumors in relation to post-menopausal estrogen therapy. *New England Journal of Medicine* **290,** 15–19.
54. Leissner, K-H., Wedel, H., Schersten, T. (1977). Comparison between the use of oral contraceptives and the incidence of surgically confirmed gallstone disease. *Scandinavian Journal of Gastroenterology* **12,** 893–6.
55. Boston Collaborative Drug Surveillance Programme (1973). Oral contraceptives and venous thromboembolic disease, surgically confirmed gall bladder disease, and breast tumours. *Lancet* **1,** 1399–1404.
56. Harvald, B., Hauge, M. (1956). A catamnestic investigation of Danish twins. *Danish Medical Bulletin* **3,** 150–8.
57. McConnell, R. B. (1966). *The Genetics of Gastrointestinal Disorders.* London, Oxford University Press.
58. Piper, J., Orrid, L. (1956). Essential familial hypercholesterolaemia: a follow-up study of 12 Danish families. *American Journal of Medicine* **21,** 34–40.
59. Bell, G. D., Lewis, B., Petrie, A., Dowling, R. H. (1973). Serum lipids in cholelithiasis: effects of chenodeoxycholic acid therapy. *British Medical Journal* **3,** 520–2.
60. Boonyapisit, S. T., Trotman, B. W., Ostrow, J. D. (1978). Unconjugated bilirubin, and the hydrolysis of conjugated bilirubin, in gall bladder bile of patients with cholelithiasis. *Gastroenterology* **74,** 70–4.

7
Pancreatitis

Discussion of the epidemiology of pancreatitis is limited by the difficulties of case ascertainment. The diagnosis of acute pancreatitis is not in doubt in patients with acute abdominal pain and a grossly raised serum amylase, and chronic pancreatitis is a sure diagnosis in patients with pancreatic calcification. In most patients diagnostic criteria are less clear, and it is impossible to calculate reliable incidence or prevalence figures. A further complication is that acute disease in some, but not all, progresses to chronic disease. If universally acknowledged criteria for disease diagnosis are used, as must be the case, then we shall as a result gain figures which are the lowest estimates of disease frequency because many patients with pancreatitis, and especially chronic pancreatitis, have symptoms and clinical findings which are suggestive but not diagnostic.

A further problem is added by the difficulty of deciding which patients have acute and which chronic disease. This is a clinical distinction and one often-used classification divides patients into those with acute disease, acute relapsing disease and chronic disease. The causes of all varieties of disease overlap and therefore the epidemiological features of pancreatitis of all varieties have much in common.

Incidence and time trends
Comparisons of figures obtained in different places and at different times is hindered by difficulty in knowing whether consistent diagnostic criteria have been applied and whether an equal degree of diagnostic effort has been made on each occasion. Figures for acute pancreatitis are probably comparable, but there is great difficulty in relating figures for chronic pancreatitis frequency made in different places because of varying diagnostic criteria.

Table 7.1 shows that taken overall there is a reasonable uniformity in the frequency of acute pancreatitis recorded in the USA and in the United Kingdom. Whether similar results would be obtained elsewhere is doubtful: thus in areas like France, where alcohol consumption is heavy, incidence rates for acute and chronic pancreatitis are likely to be high, whilst in other areas, such as parts of

130 Pancreatitis

Table 7.1 Pancreatitis

(a) Annual incidence per 100 000 population

UK: Bristol	1962–67[1]	(Acute)	5·4
Glasgow	1974[2]	(Acute)	10·0
Nottingham	1969–74[3]	(Acute)	4·8
USA, Minnesota	1960–69[4]	(Acute)	11·4
		(Chronic)	3·5

(b) Mortality per 100 000 population

UK: Bristol[1]	(Acute)	0·9
Nottingham[3]	(Acute)	0·9
England and Wales, 1969[5]	(Acute)	1·1

South India, calcific pancreatitis is common but is unassociated with alcohol intake.

Mortality rates within the United Kingdom show reasonable uniformity (Table 7.1), but there is no certainty that this uniformity would be detected elsewhere, for the same reasons as given for expecting variations in incidence. The death rate from chronic pancreatitis is very low, so much so that it cannot be used as an indirect measure of disease frequency.

Within the United Kingdom the number of deaths from acute

Table 7.2 Average number of deaths each year from acute pancreatitis in England and Wales.[6]

	Men	Women
1956–58	151	239
1959–61	185	246
1962–64	236	303
1965–67	252	307
1968–70	224	301
1971–73	268	326
1974–76	303	352

Table 7.3 Crude death rate from acute pancreatitis in the USA.

	Rate per 100 000
1955	1·0
1959–61	1·1
1965	1·3

pancreatitis has risen steadily in the last twenty years. This trend suggests an increase in the frequency of acute pancreatitis, perhaps due to a general rise in alcohol consumption in the population. The death rate is now approximately 1 per 100 000 population per year, a figure which is much the same as that recorded in the United States where death rates may also be rising slowly (Tables 7.2–3).

Support for the view that a rise in disease incidence explains the rise in death rates can be derived from a survey in Rochester, Minnesota where the frequency of both acute and chronic pancreatitis seems to have risen distinctly (Table 7.4).

Table 7.4 Average annual incidence of acute and chronic pancreatitis in Rochester, Minnesota.[4]

	1940–49		1950–59		1960–69	
	Number	Incidence*	Number	Incidence	Number	Incidence
Acute	18	6·8	46	13·7	52	11·4
Chronic	5	1·9	14	4·2	16	3·5

* Per 100 000 per year.

Geographical trends

Examination of geographical trends is complicated by the need to discriminate between cases associated with gallstones or with alcohol consumption, and those in which neither of these factors appear to operate.

Pancreatitis, acute and chronic, is common in all areas where alcohol intake is socially customary, and Table 7.4 shows the proportions of cases associated with alcohol consumption, gallstones or other (mainly unknown) factors. The strength of associations with alcohol consumption or gallstones varies greatly, and is difficult to explain. It is likely to depend in part upon the amount of alcohol consumed by the population at large, in part upon the diagnostic criteria for pancreatitis, there being possibly a greater chance of calcific disease in alcohol consumers; and in part upon the sources of the patients collected in these clinical surveys. In the absence of agreed criteria and reproducible criteria for the diagnosis of chronic pancreatitis and with the lack of general population surveys, it is hard to do more than point to the general importance of both alcohol intake and gallstones in the induction of pancreatitis. Thus in the United States, Howard and Ehrlick[15] noted that pancreatitis associated with gallbladder disease tended to be more frequent in general hospitals than in charity hospitals, but within the charity hospitals surveyed the relative frequencies of alcohol intake and gallbladder disease associated with pancreatitis varied by four-fold or more, and they were unable to explain this variation.

Table 7.5 Chronic pancreatitis: frequency of associated alcoholism and gallstones.

	Alcohol	Gallbladder disease	Other factors or unknown
France[8]	89·1	3·6	7·3
Germany[9]	11·3	19·3	69·4
Ireland[10]	7·6	41·5	50·9
Japan[11]	32·6	10·0	57·4
South Africa[12]	80·0	1·0	19·0
Switzerland[13]	61·8*	3·8*	34·3
UK[14]	4·5	31·8	63·7
USA: (i)[15]	86·2	2·8	11·0
(ii)[16]	59·2	9·5	31·3
(iii)[17]	23·3	35·0	41·7

* 1·9% of both alcohol and gallbladder disease.

Nutrition

Any evidence associating nutritional factors apart from alcohol intake with the incidence of chronic pancreatitis is fragmentary. Thus, it has been claimed that a raised protein and fat intake are significant associated factors with alcoholic disease[8,23] but this suggestion ill accords with the belief, again insecurely founded, that malnutrition predisposes to pancreatitis, and the differences noted from controls were small (Table 7.6).

Table 7.6 Dietary intake patterns in patients with chronic pancreatitis and control individuals.[8]

	Patients (55)	Control 1 (55)	Control 2* (55)
Alcohol	175	74	74
Fat	125	99	106
Protein	119	104	107
Carbohydrate	425	430	436

* Nature of control group not stated.

Clinically there has been a repeated suggestion that patients with hyperlipidaemia are prone to pancreatitis.[24] The origin of such hyperlipidaemia does not necessarily seem to be dietary for it has been ascribed to oral contraceptive use.[25] Increases in serum triglyceride levels with lactescent serum have been suggested as particular features together with prebeta-lipoproteinaemia.[26]

Associated conditions

Though a range of conditions including hypothermia, viral infections, especially mumps, acute hepatic failure,[27] penetrating duodenal ulcer, scorpion bites,[28] and pregnancy[29] (though this has been contested) have been thought to be associated with liability to acute pancreatitis, there is no evidence that these predispose to chronic disease. A small proportion of patients with chronic pancreatitis have been noted to have hypercalcaemia and hyperlipidaemia. Hypercalcaemia of any variety probably predisposes to pancreatitis, for acute pancreatitis has been associated with hypercalcaemia in multiple myeloma[30] as well as with that due to hyperparathyroidism.[31]

Drug-induced pancreatitis

Associations noted clinically have been with acute pancreatitis, and case reports have been put forward to suggest, *inter alia*, associations with corticosteroid, azathioprin, paracetamol and oral contraceptive treatment. The strength, and indeed the existence of these associations require demonstration by case-control studies. Claims for an association between diuretic treatment and acute pancreatitis have been supported by such a case-control study.[32]

Genetic factors

Recurrent pancreatitis occurs in hereditary hyperlipaemia and hyperparathyroidism. In addition relapsing pancreatitis has been described with inheritance as an autosomal dominant in several families.[33] Chronic pancreatic insufficiency also occurs in some four-fifths of children with fibrocystic disease which is inherited as an autosomal recessive.

References

1. Trapnell, J. E. and Duncan, E. H. L. (1975). Patterns of incidence in acute pancreatitis. *British Medical Journal* **2,** 179–83.
2. Irvine, C. W. (1974). Observations on acute pancreatitis. *British Journal of Surgery* **61,** 539–44.
3. Bourke, J. B. (1975). Variation in annual incidence of primary acute pancreatitis in Nottingham, 1969–74. *Lancet* **2,** 967–9.

4. O'Sullivan, J. N., Nobrega, F. T., Morlock, C. G., Brown, A. L. Jr., and Bartholomew, L. G. (1972). Acute and chronic pancreatitis in Rochester, Minnesota, 1940–1969. *Gastroenterology* **62,** 373–9.
5. *Registrar General's Statistical Review of England and Wales, 1969.* HMSO, 1971.
6. *Registrar General's Statistical Reviews of England and Wales, 1963, 1973.* HMSO, 1965, 1976. O.P.C.S. 1974, 1975, 1976 Mortality statistics England and Wales. HMSO 1977–78.
7. Mendeloff, A. I., Dunn, J. P. (1971). Digestive Diseases. Vital and Health Statistics Monographs. Cambridge, American Public Health Association, Harvard University Press.
8. Sarles, H., Sarles, J. C., Camatte, R., Muratore, R., Gaini, M., Guien, C., Pastor, J., Le Roy, F. (1965). Observations on 205 confirmed cases of acute pancreatitis, recurring pancreatitis and chronic pancreatitis. *Gut* **6,** 545–59.
9. Muller Wieland, K. (1965). Analyse der Klinik der chronischen Pankreatitis. *Zeitschrift fur clinische medizin* **158,** 371–98.
10. Fitzgerald, O., Fitzgerald, P., Fennelly, T., McMullin, J. P., Boland, S. J. (1963). A clinical study of chronic pancreatitis. *Gut* **4,** 193–216.
11. Ishii, K., Nakamura, K., Takeuchi, T., Hirayama, T. (1973). Chronic calcifying pancreatitis and pancreatic carcinoma in Japan. *Digestion* **9,** 429–37.
12. Marks, I. N., Bank, S., Louw, J. H. (1973). Chronic pancreatitis in the Western Cape. *Digestion* **9,** 447–53.
13. Amman, R. W., Hammer, B., Fumagalli, I. (1973). Chronic pancreatitis in Zurich, 1963–72. *Digestion* **9,** 404–15.
14. Howat, H. T. (1965). In: Symposium of Marseilles, April 1963: Etiology and pathological anatomy of chronic pancreatitis. Bibliotheca gastroenterologica (Basel).
15. Howard, J. H., Ehrlich, E. W. (1960). The aetiology of pancreatitis. *Annals of Surgery* **152,** 135–46.
16. White, T. T. *et al.*, quoted by Creutzfeld, W. and Schmidt, H. (1970). Aetiology and pathogenesis of chronic pancreatitis (current concepts). *Scandinavian Journal of Gastroenterology* suppl. **6,** 47–62.
17. Warren, K. W., Veidenheimer, M. (1962). Pathological considerations in the choice of operation for chronic relapsing pancreatitis. *New England Journal of Medicine* **266,** 323–9.
18. George, P. K., Banks, P. A., Pai, K. N., Ramachandran, M., Thangavelu, M., Tandon, B. N. (1971). Exocrine pancreatic function in calcific pancreatitis in India. *Gastroenterology* **60,** 858–69.
19. Zuidema, P. J. (1959). Cirrhosis and disseminated calcification of the pancreas in patients with malnutrition. *Tropical and Geographical Medicine* **11,** 70–4.
20. Shaper, A. G. (1964). Aetiology of chronic pancreatic fibrosis with calcification seen in Uganda. *British Medical Journal* **1,** 1607–9.
21. Banwell, J. G., Hutt, M. S. R., Leonard, P. J., Blackman, V., Connor, D. W., Marsden, P. D., Campbell, J. (1967). Exocrine pancreatic disease and the malabsorption syndrome in tropical Africa. *Gut* **8,** 388–401.
22. Kinnear, T. W. G. (1963). The pattern of diabetes mellitus in a Nigerian teaching hospital. *East African Medical Journal* **40,** 288–94.
23. Sarles, H. (1973). An international survey on nutrition and pancreatitis. *Digestion* **9,** 389–403.

24. Cameron, J. L., Capuzzi, D. M., Zuidema, G. D., Margolis, S. (1973). Acute pancreatitis with hyperlipemia: incidence of lipid abnormalities in acute pancreatitis. *Annals of Surgery* **177**, 483–9.
25. Davidoff, F., Tishler, S., Rosoff, C. (1973). Marked hyperlipidemia and pancreatitis associated with oral contraceptive therapy. *New England Journal of Medicine* **289**, 552–5.
26. Farmer, R. G., Winkelman, E. I., Brown, H. B., Lewis, L. A. (1973). Hyperlipoproteinemia and pancreatitis. *American Journal of Medicine* **54**, 161–5.
27. Ham, J. M., Fitzpatrick, P. (1973). Acute pancreatitis in patients with acute hepatic failure. *American Journal of Digestive Diseases* **18**, 1079–83.
28. Bartholomew, C. (1970). Acute scorpion pancreatitis in Trinidad. *British Medical Journal* **1**, 666–8.
29. Berk, J. E., Smith, B. H., Akrawi, M. M. (1971). Pregnancy pancreatitis. *American Journal of Gastroenterology* **56**, 216–26.
30. Meltzer, L. E., Palmon, F. P., Paik, Y. K., Custer, R. P. (1962). Acute pancreatitis secondary to hypercalcaemia of multiple myeloma. *Annals of Internal Medicine* **57**, 1008–12.
31. Banks, P. A., Janowitz, H. D. (1969). Some metabolic aspects of exocrine pancreatic disease. *Gastroenterology* **56**, 601–17.
32. Bourke, J. B., McIllmurray, M. B., Mead, G. M., Langman, M. J. S. (1978). Drug-associated primary acute pancreatitis. *Lancet* **1**, 706–8.
33. Whitten, D. M., Feingold, M., Eisenklam, E. J. (1968). Hereditary pancreatitis. *American Journal of Diseases of Childhood* **116**, 426–8.

Index

Alcohol
  colonic cancer 62
  oesophageal cancer 47
  pancreatitis 132
  peptic ulcer 25, 26
Angiosarcoma 70
Appendicitis 109 *et seq*
  diet 110, 111
  geographical distribution 109
  incidence 109
  predisposing factors 110
  time trends 110
Aspergillus and cancer 72

Bacteria and Crohn's disease 87
Bacterial metabolism
  colonic cancer 63
  gallstones 123
Bile acids
  colonic cancer 63
  gallstones 119
Bile duct cancer and colitis 74

Cancer 40 *et seq*
  bile duct
    associated diseases 72
    gallstones 73
  colonic 57 *et seq*
    age incidence 58
    associated disease 60
    bacterial metabolism 63
    bile acids 63
    Crohn's disease 61
    environmental factors 62
    general incidence 58
    geographical factors 57
    inheritance 60
    migrants 65
    occupation 60
    polyps 60
    sex incidence 58
    social factors 60
    time trends 60
    transit time 65
    ulcerative colitis 61

death rates
  reliability 41
gall bladder 72
  associated diseases 73
  gallstones 73
gastric 49 *et seq*
  age incidence 45, 50
  associated disease 52
  diet 54, 55
  environmental factors 53
  general incidence 50
  geographical factors 13, 19
  inheritance 53
  migrants 53
  nitrosation 55
  occupation 51
  post-operative 53
  sex incidence 50
  smoking 55
  social factors 51
  time trends 51
  trace elements 55
hepatic 69 *et seq*
  associated disease 70
  drug induced 71
  geographical factors 69, 70
  occupational factors 70
  parasitic disease 72
  toxins 72
  viral associated 71
incidence rates
  standardization 42
large intestinal 57 *et seq*
  (*see also* Colonic and Rectal)
  bacteria 63
  bile acids 63
  Crohn's disease 61
  migrants 65
  polyps 60
  transit time 65
  ulcerative colitis 61
oesophageal 42 *et seq*
  age incidence 44
  alcohol 47
  associated disease 46

Index

diet 48
fungal toxins 49
general incidence 43
geographical variation 43
histology 43
nitrosation 47, 49
occupational factors 45
sex incidence 45
smoking 48
time trends 45
trace elements 49
pancreatic 66 *et seq*
  age incidence 67
  associated disease 68
  diet 68
  general incidence 66
  geographical variation 66
  occupational and social factors 68
  sex incidence 66
  smoking 69
  time trends 67
rectal 57 *et seq*
  age incidence 58
  associated disease 60
  bacterial metabolism 63
  bile acids 63
  Crohn's disease 61
  environmental factors 62
  general incidence 59
  geographical factors 58
  inheritance 60
  occupational and social factors 60
  polyps 60
  sex incidence 58
  time trends 60
  transit time 65
  ulcerative colitis 61
small intestinal 56
  adenocarcinoma 56
  carcinoid 56
  lymphoma 56
standardized mortality ratios 4
Chronic inflammatory bowel disease
  80 *et seq*
  (*see also* Crohn's disease and
    Ulcerative colitis)
associated disease
  cancer 95
  gallstones 94
  inflammatory diseases 94
  peptic ulcer 95
Cirrhosis
  gallstones 121
  peptic ulcer 30
Crohn's disease 80 *et seq*
  (*see also* Chronic inflammatory bowel
    disease)
  age distribution 84

bacterial infection 87, 88
clustering 87
contagion 86
diet 86
ethnic variation 96
gallstones 123
geographical variation 81
incidence 80
inheritance 97, 98
sex incidence 84
socio-economic factors 85
time trends 80

Death certificate accuracy 41
Diabetes mellitus
  gallstones 122
  pancreatic cancer 68
Diet
  appendicitis 111
  Crohn's disease 86
  correlation analysis 54
  diverticular disease 106
  gallstones 120
  gastric cancer 55
  pancreatic cancer 68
  pancreatitis 132
  peptic ulcer 24
  retrospective analyses 54
  ulcerative colitis 92
Dietary fibre
  appendicitis 111
  colonic cancer 65
  diverticular disease 107
  ulcer 24
Diverticular disease 103
  age distribution 104
  associated disease 108
  autopsy frequency 104
  diet 106, 107
  geographical frequency 105
  hospital admission 106
  incidence 104
  sex incidence 104
  time trends 104, 106
  transit time 108
Drugs inducing
  gallstones 124
  pancreatitis 133
  peptic ulcer 27
Duodenal ulcer
  age distribution 18
  alcohol 25, 26
  associated disease 30
  deaths 9, 10, 15, 18
  diet 24
  drug induced 29
  ethnic variation 20
  geographical variation 12, 19

hospital admissions 16
inheritance 33
smoking 25
socio-economic factors 21
time trends 14

Fungal toxins and liver cancer 72

Gallstones 114 *et seq*
  autopsy frequency 115
  diet 120
  drug induced 124
  ethnic variation 2, 117
  general incidence 115
  geographical incidence 117, 118
  haemolysis 122
  hepatic cirrhosis 121
  inheritance 125
  pancreatitis 132
  predisposing disease 121 *et seq*
  pregnancy 116
  social factors 119
  time trends 116
Gastric ulcer
  age distribution 18
  alcohol 25, 26
  associated disease 30
  cancer liability 53
  deaths 9, 10, 15, 18
  diet 24 *et seq*
  drug induced 27 *et seq*
  ethnic variation 20
  geographical variation 12, 19
  hospital admissions 16
  inheritance 33
  smoking 25
  socio-economic factors 21
  time trends 14
General epidemiology 1 *et seq*
  admission rates 1, 6
  autopsy surveys 10, 41
  death rates 5, 10
  incidence rates 2, 42
  standardization 3, 42
Geographical incidence
  Crohn's disease 81
  diverticular disease 104
  gallstones 117
  gastric cancer 50
  hepatic cancer 69
  large intestinal cancer 57
  oesophageal cancer 44
  pancreatic cancer 66
  pancreatitis 131
  peptic ulcer 13
  ulcerative colitis 90

Hepatic cirrhosis
  gallstones 121
  hepatic cancer 70
Hospital admission statistics 6

Infection
  Crohn's disease 86
  gallstones 123
  ulcerative colitis 93
Inheritance
  cancer
    colonic 60
    gastric 53
    rectal 60
  Crohn's disease 97, 98
  duodenal ulcer 33
  gallstones 125
  gastric ulcer 33
  pancreatitis 133
Intestinal transit time
  appendicitis 110
  colon cancer 65
  diverticular disease 108

Lymphoma, intestinal 56

Migrants
  colonic cancer 40, 65
  gallstones 120
  gastric cancer 40
Morbidity rates 2
  (*see also* Incidence rates for individual diseases)
Mortality rates 3, 5
  cancer 41

Nitrites
  gastric cancer 55
Nitrosamines
  gastric cancer 55
  oesophageal cancer 47, 49

Obesity and gallstones 124
Occupation
  Crohn's disease 85
  gastric cancer 51
  hepatic cancer 70
  large intestinal cancer 60
  oesophageal cancer 45
  peptic ulcer 21
Occupational mortality 5
Oral contraceptives
  gallstones 124
  hepatic tumours 71

Pancreatitis 129 *et seq*
  alcohol 132
  associated disease 132

diet 132
drug induced 133
gallstones 132
geographical variation 131
incidence 129
inheritance 133
mortality 130
time trends 129
Peptic ulcer 9 *et seq*
 (*see also* Duodenal and gastric ulcer)
 age distribution 18
 alcohol 25, 26
 associated disease 30
 deaths 9, 10, 15, 18
 diet 24
 drug induced 27
 general incidence 9, 12
 geographical variation 12, 19
 hospital admissions 16
 incidence 17
 inheritance 33
 psychological factors 35
 smoking 25
 socio-economic factors 21
 time trends 14
Pernicious anaemia and gastric cancer 52
Plant toxins and gastric cancer 72
Polyps and large bowel cancer 60
Prevalence rates 3

Regional enteritis (*see* Crohn's disease)

Smoking
 gastric cancer 55
 oesophageal cancer 48
 pancreatic cancer 49
 peptic ulcer 25
Social class
 Crohn's disease 85
 gallstones 119
 gastric cancer 52
 large intestinal cancer 60
 peptic ulcer 22
Standardization
 cancer incidence 41
 mortality rates 3
 mortality ratios 4

Time trends
 Crohn's disease 81
 gallstones 116
 gastric cancer 52
 intestinal cancer 62
 pancreatic cancer 67
 peptic ulcer 14
 rectal cancer 62
 ulcerative colitis 83
Toxins
 fungal 49
 hepatic cancer 72
 plant 72
Trace elements
 gastric cancer 55
 oesophageal cancer 49
Tropics
 hepatic cancer 69
 oesophageal cancer 43
 peptic ulcer 13, 23
 ulcerative colitis 90

Ulcerative colitis (*see also* Chronic inflammatory bowel disease)
 age incidence 91
 associated diseases 94
 auto-immunity 93
 cancer in 95
 diet 92
 ethnic variation 96
 genetic factors 97
 incidence 89
 infection 93
 sex incidence 91
 socio-economic factors 92
 time trends 90
Ulcer, peptic (*see* Duodenal ulcer, Gastric ulcer, Peptic ulcer)

Viruses and Crohn's disease 86
Vitamin deficiency and oesophageal cancer 48

Yersinia and Crohn's disease 88